cease

cease

A MEMOIR OF LOVE, LOSS AND DESIRE

LYNETTE LOEPPKY

OOLICHAN BOOKS
FERNIE, BRITISH COLUMBIA, CANADA
2014

Library and Archives Canada Cataloguing in Publication

Loeppky, Lynette Dawn, 1966-, author

           Cease / Lynette Dawn Loeppky.

ISBN 978-0-8892-309-9 (pbk.)

           1. Loeppky, Lynette Dawn, 1966-. 2. Lesbianism. 3. Lesbians—
Biography. I. Title

HQ75.4.L64A3 2014   306.76'63092   C2014-905869-1

We gratefully acknowledge the financial support of the Canada Council for the Arts, the British Columbia Arts Council through the BC Ministry of Tourism, Culture, and the Arts, and the Government of Canada through the Canada Book Fund, for our publishing activities.

Published by
Oolichan Books
P.O. Box 2278
Fernie, British Columbia
Canada V0B 1M0

www.oolichan.com

Printed in Canada

For
Cecile Georgina Kaysoe
May 5, 1952 – March 21, 2005

Author's Note

Cease is a work of creative nonfiction. Many parts of the story have been fictionalized to varying degrees for literary effect.

In an effort to protect privacy, there are people who were important in Cecile's life and in mine, including family members, who do not appear at all. As well, some names have been changed and, in some instances, multiple individuals have been condensed into one character. All descriptions and representations of people are not to be considered definitive but only a subjective interpretation filtered through the lens of personal perspective.

Events and locations have been recreated from memory and should not be understood as literal in all cases. Dialogue does not represent word-for-word transcripts. *Cease* is told from a single narrative perspective and is true only insomuch as any one person's interpretation of experience is true to that person.

I do not claim to tell the definitive story of Cecile's life or death, or presume to speak on her behalf in any way. The story, the experiences and the words are mine alone.

Every person wishes for a subtle assassin, the natural magic of a perfectly arranged end.

Restlessness, Aritha van Herk

I close my eyes and see her falling. Again. Her foot pushes the ladder and she topples, weightless against a blur of blue sky, ground rushing up.

When I open my eyes, her falling stops.

But as soon as I close my eyes, there she is again, in her brown coveralls, plaid blue-red work shirt, tool belt lifted by the push of air, baseball cap spiralling. Her blonde hair is flattened from the cap but flipped up at the edges and spread like wings. She hugs her arms to her chest, refuses to reach toward earth.

A gust of wind, she said later, just as she'd reached the top of the ladder and gripped the shingles tighter, ready to heave them onto the slope of the barn roof. A gust pushed the ladder and she found herself standing perfectly vertical on the top rung.

"I can't break my glasses," she thought and dropped the shingles, straight down. She pushed with her feet, away from the barn, away from the watering trough, determined not to break a leg, or a hand. "Relax," she told herself. She closed her eyes and let herself fall.

That was five years ago.

I stare up at the edge of the barn roof, then over to the depression in the dirt where her shoulder hit first. She walked gingerly for days after that, hunched forward. A broken rib, according to her self-diagnosis. Probably several broken ribs.

"But I didn't break my glasses, or my hands." She tried to smile. "I need my hands."

The roof slope on the north side where she fell is steep, much steeper than on the south side where an overhang reaches out from the roof and is supported by three rough-hewn poles. The overhang has taken the worst beating by winter winds, wide swaths of particleboard cleared of shingles.

I should patch the roof, but whenever I think about getting out the ladder, I see her again, standing on the top rung. And then she is falling.

The snow has melted, the ground getting spongier under my feet as it warms. I collect the scattered shingle pieces and throw them into the middle of the small corral. I called Stan, who lives three miles south, to bring his Bobcat and move the pile of cow shit from the corral and out behind the barn to the edge of the gully. Bobcat teeth have scarred the damp dirt and are overlaid with the imprints of Griff's large paws. Noddy trots along behind Griff, but he's so light he doesn't leave a mark.

My boots make slurpy, suctioning sounds. Griff and Noddy are circling, noses down. The dirt is scraggly with the remains of dried weeds. Melting snow has gathered into a large puddle in the middle of the corral. There's a drainage channel but it clogs up when we get a big melt. I'll have to get the shovel, maybe the pickaxe.

Griff stops his corral inspection to keep a closer eye on me. *Time for a walk? Are we going soon?* He's the size and shape of a lab with a dark chocolate undercoat and fine silvery overcoat—a Wirehaired Griffon, a bird-dog with a love of water. He'll fling himself into a creek or pond with joyful abandon. Took a magpie right out of the air once. We were up on the dead-end road and a magpie was coming in for a landing on a bush. I heard a squawk and turned. The magpie was gasping, crushed in Griff's jaws.

Griff drops his nose to the ground again, inspecting the seam where the barn wall meets the dirt under the overhang. He's hoping for the scurry of a mouse, the dart of a gopher. His nose is all concentration, his back end wiggling. "A big, happy boy," the vet calls him.

Noddy has his nose down too. He's Griff's little sidekick, part Yorkie and part poodle, he has a curly peach-coloured coat, more poodle than Yorkie. Nod follows Griff's lead, more or less, but doesn't pay much attention to birds—unless one of the chickens has flapped its way up to the top of the mesh that surrounds the run. A Buff Orpington, or a Red Rock. The Silkies are too small. Their fluffy wings can barely get them off the ground.

I'd never seen a Silkie before we moved out here and Cec's sister brought us half a dozen as a farm-warming gift. We hadn't planned on having animals, hadn't really planned anything. We bought the farm as a weekend getaway from the pressure of two full-time careers, hers in freight forwarding, mine in sales. But when Cec's sister opened the box and we saw the little trembling balls of black fluff, our weekend retreat turned into a hobby farm.

The Silkie hens turned out to be determined setters and fiercely protective mother hens. Except for "Stew," the lone rooster who was a scaredy-chicken. He would run squawking at the slightest disturbance and burrow under the hens at night.

Cec wanted to let them roam in the yard. She liked the idea of free ranging.

"No." I planted my feet, folded my arms. "Too tempting for the coyotes."

"We'd lock them up at night," Cec said, pointing at the white shed that we'd just emptied of tools and filled with straw.

"It'd be like sending out dinner invitations."

I expected Cec to shrug, or pretend she hadn't heard me. Surprisingly she acquiesced and got to work digging postholes.

The mesh we nailed to the posts was four feet high, low enough that we'd occasionally see Griff standing transfixed, his face lifted, waiting for the dumb chicken teetering on the top of the wire to launch itself into the yard. Noddy would be right beside him, yapping and lunging. Charlie, our Nova Scotia Duck Toller, would hang back waiting for the chase.

For a Duck Toller, Charlie showed surprisingly little interest in birds. But then we weren't a hundred percent sure she was a Duck Toller. A guy Cec worked with had found her abandoned in a park. He'd thought she was male and named her Charlie. We tried calling her Carly, but without success. Charlie stuck.

I toss the last of the shingles onto the pile and head for the corral gate. Griff charges toward the house, Noddy chasing after him. Charlie is already waiting on the back stoop. She wants to be sure I get the gun from the back porch. That's the sure sign we're heading out.

I fill the clip with bullets, shove it into my pocket, and rest the butt of the twenty-two against my shoulder as I step out onto the cement stoop by the back door, which is leaning slightly and chipped at the edges.

The dogs take off, racing, Noddy always in the rear, his legs too short to keep up. At the end of the driveway they veer right onto the dead-end dirt road that fades into a set of tire tracks and eventually devolves even further into a grassy trail along the top ridge of the gully.

I like the scuff of my steel-toed boots on the packed earth; the scrub grass like a carpet, an expanse of grassland textured with sage and a burst of crocuses for two days every May.

"Pick up your feet!" Cec would say. It's as though she's right beside me—her confident stride, her alertness. She would always see the coyote before I did, sometimes before the dogs.

The slope of prairie into the gully looks gradual but the embankment is steep and the creek farther away than it seems, and wider, and deeper. The bottom of the gully is like a flat-bottomed boat, lots of room for the curving meander of the creek, or what's left of it. The property line of our forty acres, a long narrow strip of land, extends down into the gully and three-quarters of the way across—our bottom pasture.

The dogs careen down the embankment toward the creek, their legs flying so fast I expect to see one of them trip in a gopher hole. They never do. I call after them, "Not too far," but my words are whipped away by the wind.

I call again. Not even a twitch of an ear.

I'm jogging after them, watching for badger holes.

Griff has reached the creek, Noddy right behind him. There are coyote dens along the embankment. My eyes scan the rocks and patches of dry grass. A coyote would snatch up Noddy in a wink. I'm a terrible shot. I couldn't hit the broad side of a barn never mind a coyote.

If only I could whistle. Cec could let loose a piercing blast and the dogs would come running back. When I try to whistle all that leaves my lips is spit and air. Cec would double over laughing.

"Come on buddies. Come on back." I try for friendly, cheerful. "I'll give you a treat!" Usually that works. "Treeeat…" Nothing.

All three have their noses to the ground. Watching them, I realize they're trying to pick up a scent.

"Griffeeee."

Griff lifts his head and looks back over his shoulder at me.

"Aaaahhhh…" I yell until I am hoarse. I lower the butt of the gun to the ground and sink onto the dried remains of last year's sage.

They think I've brought them out here to find her.

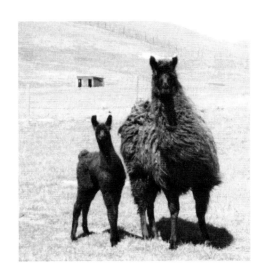

"Were there signs?"

Sunday, February 27

I drove Cec into Emergency in Calgary on a Sunday morning, late February. We stood in line, Cec steadying herself against me until the intake nurse nodded, and we inched forward.

"Name?" The nurse lifted her pen.

Cec clutched my arm tighter.

"Cecile Kaysoe," I said.

"Your name or hers?"

"Her name."

"She's the one presenting today?"

"Yes."

"The reason you've come to Emergency?"

"She has pain, severe pain, in her…"

The nurse looked up. "I need to hear it from her," she said, jabbing her pen in Cec's direction.

Cec tried but her words were indecipherable. The nurse leaned forward, "Can you speak up?"

I squeezed Cec's hand and glared. "No, she can't. She can barely stand."

The nurse's face was round and soft—plump cheeks, large turquoise-rimmed glasses, loosely curlered hair—but her words were clipped. "Where's the pain?"

"Her back," I said, nudging Cec to the side and stepping in front of the window.

"A walk-in clinic will be faster. There's one just…"

"She's been to a clinic."

"Emergency should be your very last recourse."

"It is. We've exhausted all other options."

"It could be a while before anyone can see you."

"We'll wait."

The farmyard sags. The barn, the sheds, the chicken runs look grey, sunken, haggard. The buoyancy of the place has settled into a melancholic contemplation. Or is it just me, my own lethargy.

Canny, our quarter horse mare, stands at the gate to the top pasture chewing a single strand of alfalfa, her intelligent brown eyes following me. She'll let me get within an arm's length then toss her head and prance out of reach, punishing me for taking Cec away.

I miss the eerily human bleat of the goats, and I'm glad I didn't get rid of all the chickens. I had one of our neighbours come pick up the Silkies, the Buff Orpingtons, the Jersey Giants, the Wyandottes, the Cochins, the Welsummers. I kept back half a dozen Red Rocks. They lay large brown eggs, and if I could bring myself to eat them they're also good meat birds. But I can't imagine plucking the brown feathers or sitting down to a plate of familiar plump breasts, crisp browned thighs.

I fill my pockets with alfalfa cubes from a bucket just inside the barn door. Canny perks her ears. She knows.

I settled us into seats that allowed me a full view of the Emergency admitting window and the nurse-sentry in her flowered shirt. I fired a stream of telepathic reminders in her direction. Noddy was waiting in the car in the small parking lot across from the Emergency entrance. I needed to check on him and add money to the meter.

I kept my eyes trained on the intake nurse—a steady

gaze, no glowering, although the flush of my cheeks must have given me away.

The first thing Cec said to me that morning was, "I can't do this anymore."

"I'll take you in?"

She nodded.

About bloody time! I thought. What I said was, "Chores?"

"You'll have to do them."

I pulled on my coveralls and rushed through chores, as fast as I could, my mind trying to shake the fog of morning. Cec was out of the shower and packing an overnight bag when I came back in.

"Should we take him?" Noddy was prancing at my heels. He knew we were going somewhere, didn't matter where, and he wanted to come.

"I don't know. You decide."

I hated it when she said that. Whatever decision I made was guaranteed to be the wrong one. But this time her irritation was dulled by exhaustion and a struggle to form words. For the first time in our eight and a half years, she didn't seem to have an opinion.

"Yes," I said to Nod, "you can come." He ran to the back door, wriggling, scratching.

"What can I take?"

Cec handed me her leather backpack and picked up her purse.

"I can take that too," I said, reaching. She shook her head. Her purse bulged and thumped against her hip. She was wearing her favorite cords, deep red and frayed at the edges, and a cream-coloured Ralph Lauren turtleneck. With her black ball cap pulled down over her eyes, wisps of blonde hair peeking out from under, she looked part innocent child, part wise crone.

She set her purse down in the back entrance and pulled on her burgundy leather jacket. She was moving slowly but with the same contained self-assurance as the first time I saw her standing in the reception area at work. She was wearing a cream turtleneck that day too, I think, but her hair was lighter then, a bright blonde, almost white.

I stepped out the back door onto the cement stoop just ahead of her. The air was cool. I could hear Cec's voice in my head: *You could have brought the car around.*

I should have.

You just don't think! Her voice again.

She was almost right. I lived in my mind, inside a stream of contemplation and analysis. When I went outside, my inclination was to sit on the edge of the deck and wonder at the clouds. When Cec stepped out the door, she saw the grass that needed mowing, weeds in the flower beds, a fence waiting to be fixed. She'd be adding chores to her mental list as she headed for the barn to get her pitchfork. "You coming?" I was always three steps behind, ten seconds late.

Cec picked her way carefully across the gravel. The yard was patchy with snow from a mid-February melt, the top layer crispy from melting and re-freezing. She stopped at the edge of the grass, took a long look at the row of bony cow rumps in the small corral, their noses buried in hay. Canny and Chase stood at the gate to the top pasture, their ears perked, the llamas a careful distance back.

Noddy was scratching at the gravel, anxious for the car door to open. Cec waited until I got into the driver's seat before she eased herself onto the back seat. She could stretch her legs better back there, adjust her position. If she sat for too long, shards of pain would shoot up her spine. I was already steeling myself.

Cec didn't say anything as we drove down the driveway. She watched out the window, a last look at the llamas, the horses, the cows, the protective cluster of buildings, the stacks of bales. Usually she would call out, "See ya bubbas!" But today she sat with her hands in her lap, studying the contours of the top pasture, the angles of receding rooftops, the certainty of the fences.

The waiting room was about half full: several sets of parents with small children, an elderly East Indian couple who sat very still staring straight ahead, a large man in a work shirt and work boots his head tilted back against the wall, mouth open, eyes closed.

Cec leaned against me, briefly. She straightened. I lifted my arm to put it around her but she murmured, "No."

One guy walked past the lineup to the nurse behind the glass. He leaned forward, one hand on his chest. Immediate action. The intake nurse called for another nurse who ushered him into a small side room and had him sit in a chair, roll up his sleeve. She closed the door.

I sat stiffly, willing my knees not to jiggle. I knew the tremors would bother Cec.

"Are you hungry?" I asked.

She shook her head, no. "But maybe I should eat something."

"I'm going to see if I can find a sandwich and check on Nod. What can I bring you?"

"Egg salad, if they have it."

"You'll be okay?"

She nodded.

"Call me if they come for you."

Nothing.

"I won't be long."

It was a relief to stand, finally, to be in motion. I felt guilty. Didn't seem fair that I could just get up and walk away from her pain but she couldn't.

I'd listened to her pace, middle of the night, from the bedroom through the living room to the kitchen.

"It's like I have a hot dagger in my back," she said. "Can't lie flat. Can't sit. Can't stand still."

When she did try to lie down, any movement of the bed would send pain shooting up her spine. Finally she couldn't stand it anymore. She cleared a space upstairs and made a bed for herself on the floor.

"Can't bear it when you move," she said gruffly.

But the futon was low to the floor, and the stairs were steep.

I was a bit slow, but I finally realized that I should be the one sleeping upstairs—let her have our bed and the whole of the main floor for her middle-of-the-night pacing.

The futon was lumpy. I flopped from side to side, listening, monitoring. Her footsteps would stop and I'd hold my breath, wait for her pacing to resume.

I could imagine her, leaning against the table, resting her weight on the heels of her hands, rocking back and forth. If I asked whether there was anything I could do she would wave me away. "It's easier when you're not here."

The Emergency doors slid open and I braced against the wind, pulled my collar up around my ears. This was going to be a long day for Noddy. Maybe I shouldn't have brought him. I opened the car door and he scrambled out. I clipped on his leash. He sniffed the car tire and lifted his leg.

Noddy was eight weeks old when Cec went to pick him up. She'd always wanted a tiny dog, she said, a really little one, the kind you could carry in your purse. Yes, she was aware that we already had a farm full of animals but that was the whole point: one more wouldn't make a difference. His plump belly fit in the palm of Cec's hand, tiny paws dangling.

"Cecile Kaysoe?" A nurse in navy scrubs was holding a clipboard against her hip, scanning the waiting room.

"Would you like a wheelchair?" she asked as we made our way toward her, slowly.

No, Cec shook her head, her brow furrowed with determination.

The nurse led us to a bed at the end of hall, handed Cec a hospital gown, and pulled the curtain around as she left. Cec shrugged out of her jacket and pulled her turtleneck over her head. I helped her undo her bra, untie her shoes.

"My slippers," she said. "They're in the bag."

She perched on the edge of the bed as I pulled her slippers onto her cold feet.

"I can't lie flat," she said, looking at the bed. I was searching for a way to raise the back of the bed when a female voice called, "Hello?" from the other side of the curtain. A nurse with dark shoulder-length hair in navy scrubs pulled it back.

"My name is Diana. And you're…Cecile?"

Cec nodded. "Can the back go up?" She pointed at the bed. Diana pressed a button and the back raised slowly.

"And you are…" She turned to me, "her sister?"

"I'm her partner."

"Partner," Diana said. She didn't seem surprised. I was glad she hadn't asked whether Cec was my mother. We got that sometimes.

Diana pulled up a rolling stool and sat with her clipboard on her knee. "Last name spelled K-a-y-s-o-e?"

Cec nodded, her shoulders slumped. It seemed to me that she was crumbling. I settled into a chair on the far side of the bed.

"When did the pain start?" Diana asked. I leaned forward. I wanted to hear Cec's answer. Whenever I'd asked, she had just shrugged.

"About two months ago," Cec said, "or maybe two-and-a-half. Before Christmas."

Before Christmas. That meant that she was in pain when we went to Vancouver.

"Where did you first feel the pain?"

Cec pressed the right side of her abdomen.

"Was it sharp, or dull?"

"Dull, at first."

"Constant or intermittent?"

"Intermittent. At first."

I'm moving lumber, two-by-sixes that are twelve feet long, and one-inch spruce slabs, from behind the small corral to a growing pile in front of the barn. Every time Cec took the truck to town she would bring home more fence posts and one-inch slabs of spruce. If it had been up to me, we would have stacked all the wood in one location, preferably inside the barn so it wouldn't get wet. I suggested this to Cec. She pretended she hadn't heard me and started another pile.

Grass has grown up around the stacks and I have to wrench the bottom boards free. Some are rotten. I throw these into the back of the half-ton. I'll take them to the dump in Linden. The burning pit is about fifteen feet deep and just as wide, gouged into the side of a small hill. If the dump guy is doing a burn when I get there, I'll park the truck at a distance, then walk as close as I can and hurl the boards in. Another couple steps and I could fling myself in. Not that I've been tempted. But it would be a quick and painless way to go, relatively speaking.

The worst was watching her grinding jaw, her clenched fists, the perpetual furrow in her brow. I try to keep those images out of my mind. Closing my eyes doesn't help, but lugging around these boards does, in a way. Except that I can still hear her voice, scolding: *You're wasting your time, hauling that wood around.*

I keep lifting, sorting, stacking. It's my farm now. I get to make the decisions. The more physically exhausted I am, the less the echo of her criticism grates.

It's harder to ignore the questions that keep spinning. I work until I'm sweating, but I can't stop wondering. *When did she know she was sick? Were there signs?*

I can hear her. *The reason you didn't notice is that you were walking around with your Aquarian head in the clouds.*

I probably was. But what was there to notice?

She stopped drinking chai. *Was that a sign?*

Cec was the one who introduced me to chai, the spiced black tea that she simmered on the stove until the house filled with the scent of cloves, pepper, ginger. Later she discovered the chai latte at Starbucks—with an extra pump of the sweet, spicy syrup, no foam.

Then, out of the blue, Cec announced that she wasn't going to drink chai anymore. Too sweet, she said, and hard on her stomach. It wasn't good for me, either. I should stop drinking it too.

At the time Cec's pronouncement pissed me off, the way she said it, in her executive-decision voice.

Was her sudden sensitivity to chai a symptom?

The only other possible sign was that she seemed more tired than usual, especially as we got closer to Christmas.

In mid-November she said, "Let's not exchange gifts this year."

"None at all? Not even one?"

We never put up a tree, the ornaments were too great a temptation for the cats, but every year one of us would pull out our wooden Christmas calendar in the shape of a house. The calendar sat on a cedar chest in the living room and had become our "tree." Cec was always the first to pile presents.

"I'm exhausted," she said. "Besides, there's nothing we need. What could we possibly give each other that we don't already have?"

I nodded, although I didn't actually believe her.

"I have to go to Vancouver, right before Christmas, to supervise a loading," she said. "Why don't you come with me? It can be our present to each other. We'll stay a couple extra days, make a holiday of it."

I arranged for time off. She booked a room at the Listel Hotel on Robson, because she thought I'd like the artwork, and because we could step out the front door into the crush of the Robson Street shopping crowd.

We arrived in Vancouver in the middle of the afternoon and headed out to walk the streets, breathe in the ocean air. Maybe we'd go down to the waterfront. The day was damp and cool, with a wet drizzle, not a breath of wind. Shoppers were out in full force. Only four days till Christmas.

Cec wandered in and out of shops without purpose or intent. I trailed a few steps behind, close enough that I wouldn't lose her. I watched as she lifted the sleeve of a sweater to feel for percentage of natural fibre. She didn't check the price. She wasn't really shopping.

I trudged behind her out of a brightly lit FCUK into the dark damp of milling bodies. The hard tip of a pointed toe bumped her heel. She barely noticed. We walked around the lineup outside the crepe window. There were four crepe makers in front of four windows open to the street. They poured batter and smoothed it perfectly thin and almost round. I wanted a crepe, with cinnamon and brown sugar like my mother used to make. But Cec wasn't slowing. And besides, there was something else I wanted more.

The ring Cec had given me had fallen off my finger in the middle of a deepwater workout. I had felt the odd sensation of its release as a piece of the band broke, then confirmed its absence with my thumb. The ring was gone.

I didn't have my glasses on, but when I squinted and looked straight down through the twelve feet of water I saw a small round dot at the bottom of the pool. I took a deep breath and dove. Didn't make it to the bottom the first time. Tried again. This time I got to the bottom but the water played tricks on my near-sighted eyes. One more time. My fingertip touched the edge and flipped the thin shimmer toward my hand. As I swam to the top, I could feel the sharp edges where a piece of the band had broken away.

"We can get it fixed," Cec said, holding the ring up to the light.

"I'd rather get a new one."

Cec had given me the ring our first Christmas together. We'd ripped through a big stack of presents and were sitting on the floor in a sea of wrapping paper when Cec handed me a small black box. I sensed, from the look in her eyes, that the box held a ring—the one that I would wear on the fourth finger of my left hand. I felt suddenly inadequate. We hadn't talked about rings. I hadn't bought her one.

I pushed up the lid of the box. My first thought was "chunky," but I didn't say it. I looked up and smiled. Her eyes were expectant. She reached for the box, took the ring, and slid it onto my finger.

Just a few nights before as I'd been brushing my teeth while Cec was watching the Golf Channel, I'd been wishing that I hadn't moved in with her so quickly. Classic U-Haul syndrome. We'd had dinner together twice before I left on a three-week trip to Europe. When I got back, I'd pretty much moved in.

She was still a smoker then, and I wasn't keen on living in a smoky house. She'd said she would smoke outside, that she wanted to quit anyway. But she liked to have a cigarette when she was working in the basement, and she liked to smoke while she was getting ready in the morning. I would remind her that I hadn't asked, she had offered. She would butt out and promise again. But it was fall, getting cooler, and this was her house.

My shoes were resting on her doormat, my clothes in her closet, her pictures on the walls. I was sleeping on her mattress, eating off her dishes. I'd given away my second-hand couch, my cheap university-student dishes. I'd kept a frying pan, packed my books into boxes. And now I found myself standing in front of her bathroom mirror, using her toothpaste, answering her queries: *When will you be home for dinner? Who were you talking to? Going to bed already?*

The other day she'd said, "What kept you?" when I got home from work a little later than usual.

"I had to wait for Syncrude to send a change order."

"You could have called."

"I'm sorry." The words were a reflex. As soon as I said them, I wanted to take them back. I wasn't sorry.

I sat down at the table and chewed cold pork chop and sweet potato without tasting. I cleared the table, washed the dishes, swept the kitchen floor. I waited for Cec to open her laptop before I went into the living room and turned on the TV.

I was giving her the benefit of the doubt, because she was fourteen years older than me and because she had been married, and divorced, and had recently left another seven-year relationship. I was letting her take the lead, and mad at myself for doing it.

But the thought of moving out made me tired—the energy a move would require, the starting over, having to face her outrage, her pronouncements on my inability to commit. Maybe I was too young. I'd just turned thirty. I'd never been in a serious relationship. She would say that if I wanted to leave, I should go.

But I wasn't ready. Not yet.

I could imagine moving out of her house, but not out of her bed.

I liked pulling off my jeans in the darkness of her cool bedroom, crawling under the covers, falling asleep on her sagging mattress while she watched golf, or tennis, then surfacing slowly to the muffled sound of her steps across the carpet, the shush as she pulled her arms out of her sleeves, the weight of her body sinking onto the mattress, her hand on my hip, the heat of her skin, the insistence of her desire.

She said waking me like that made her feel like a child molester.

"I like it when you wake me." And I wanted her to keep waking me. So I smiled as she slid the ring onto the fourth finger of my left hand. It was gold with two horizontal strands, a top and a bottom. There was a pattern, like waves, etched into both strands and underneath, small bands that held the two pieces together. A clunky symbolism. Too overt. And too late to say so.

Cec didn't ask why I wanted a new ring instead of getting the old one fixed. She just said, "We can look for one in Vancouver."

I was keeping my eyes open for jewelry shops as we wound our way through the crowd. The hot dog man was his own island, a line of customers curled around him like a seawall. I wanted a frankfurter. Not because I was hungry. It was the smell of fried onions, the sound of sizzling, the blackened skins splitting open.

Cec's cell rang. She said, "Hello," as I pushed open the door to a small jewelry store with bars on the windows. We stepped the two steps down into a small rectangular room with display cases of rings, watches, and earrings along three walls.

Cec was laughing, "Yeah, yeah, the worst case...we might have to look at another carrier...push back delivery, yes...no, I confirmed with Steve. He said...yes, that's right he'll be there..."

It wasn't what she said but the way she said it, the tease in her voice. The guy at the other end couldn't see the tilt of her head, but I could.

Let her flirt. We had an agreement. If either of us ever wanted to sleep with someone else, we'd tell the other first. I was pretty sure she'd keep her word.

Cec flipped her phone shut and came to stand beside me. The new ring would not be expensive. It would not have a stone. No overt symbolism.

"What do you think?" I held up a gold band. She nodded in that contemplative way that said she wasn't convinced.

"How about that one?" she said to the woman behind the counter. "Or that one?" The woman brought out the rings that Cec had pointed at and set them on the counter. One was silver with an intricate pattern reminiscent of leaves and swirls, the other gold with small etchings.

"I want something simple, no patterns."

Cec leaned over the display case. I couldn't tell whether she had retreated into her thoughts or was studying the rings. Her silence didn't seem stony. She didn't seem mad. I couldn't tell what she was thinking.

Cec's cell phone rang again. As she pulled it out of her purse, she said, "Whichever one you like. You're the one that will have to wear it."

That was it?! I was sure she'd actually care.

I thought about saying, "Forget the ring!" But then we'd have to have the argument. She would say I was being overly sensitive. And maybe I was.

I heard Cec laugh. Her sister Lora was calling to let us know that Noddy was doing fine. I held up another ring, one with three strands of different colours of gold so subtle I could barely see the nuance until I looked closely under a bright light. Cec had said goodbye and was standing at my elbow. I held up the ring with the three colours of gold. She shrugged.

Maybe she was upset because I didn't want to get the other ring fixed? Maybe her disinterest was a part of her objection to anything romantic? She hated sentimentality, wouldn't let me call her "honey" or "sweetie" or "dear." Too cliché. Too sticky-sweet. She abhorred Valentine's Day, refused to buy flowers or a card. Maybe she didn't care because getting a new ring was my idea, not hers.

"I'll take this one," I said to the saleswoman. Two

hundred and twenty-nine dollars plus tax. Cec paid with her credit card. The saleswoman put the ring into a black box and I stuck it in my pocket. It was too big for my finger. I'd have to get it sized.

When we got back to the hotel room, Cec opened her laptop and sat staring at the screen while it booted up.

I'm not sure why I asked her. Maybe it was the slump of her shoulders or the nine-hundred-thread-count Egyptian cotton sheets on the king-size bed. The duvet was a pile of clouds.

When she came to bed, she reached for me under the covers and I wriggled closer. I whispered, "It's been a long time, Babe."

The last time we'd made love was Remembrance Day three years ago. She'd left the next morning on a business trip to St. John's, Newfoundland.

"I know."

"Any idea…when?" I rarely asked anymore.

"I think I'm getting closer." She kissed my forehead. "But not tonight."

"And the pain got worse?" Diana had filled two pages with notes and was starting a third.

Cec nodded.

"When was that?"

"Over the Christmas holidays."

"Was it still a sharp pain?"

"Sometimes. More like bad gas. I felt bloated."

"Were you having a lot of gas?"

Cec glanced at me before she nodded.

"Anything else?"

"Trouble sleeping."

"Because of the pain?"

"I can't lie flat."

"Nausea?"

"Sometimes. No appetite. I eat two mouthfuls and I'm full."

She had barely touched her Christmas dinner. I had wondered but hadn't said anything.

"Early satiety," Diana said as she scribbled.

"And more tired than usual."

What Cec didn't tell Diana was that even before the pain started, she rarely slept. Cec's work area was just a few steps from the bedroom door and even though I told her it didn't bother me if she kept working after I went to bed, she rarely did. Instead she'd lie awake, for hours, listening to the muffled moos of the mama cows, their grunts as they lowered their bellies to the ground, the moan of the wind. She'd wait for the belch of the furnace to huff itself up, the initial thump loud enough to jerk her awake if she had managed to fall asleep.

By five she'd be up, checking her email. She was the national manager of Oil and Energy for an international freight-forwarding company. A staff of nine reported to her and she handled all the oversized shipments personally. Her email was constantly filled with specifications for shipments to Kazakhstan, Turkey, Chile; questions about maximum weights and dims; requests for available ship dates.

"Okay," Diana said getting up, "a doctor will be in soon to see you. I'm going to get an IV started. We need to get some fluids into you. You're pretty dehydrated. Would you like some morphine?"

Cec looked at me. "Do I want morphine?"

"Yes, you do," I said, surprised at her hesitation.

"She wants morphine," I said to Diana. "Nothing else has worked."

"I don't like drugs." Cec's voice was weak, barely audible.

"But you've been trying to get—"

"You were prescribed Naproxen." Diana checked her notes. "And OxyContin. You said that neither of those touched the pain?"

Cec stared at her blankly. "Yes. Okay."

"Okay to the morphine?"

Cec nodded.

Why had she resisted in the first place?

Diana returned a few minutes later with a transparent pouch of fluid, a smaller pouch of clear liquid, and an IV needle.

"Are you right-handed?"

Cec nodded.

Diana pulled on a pair of plastic gloves, lifted Cec's left hand, and wrapped a tourniquet below her elbow.

"Relax," she said. "Take a deep breath."

Cec closed her eyes. Diana pushed the needle into the back of Cec's hand. Cec grimaced.

Diana withdrew the needle. "Sorry," she said. "I didn't get it. It's as though your veins seize up when they sense the needle. Take another deep breath." Cec reached for my hand. Diana inserted the tip again. Cec clenched her jaw but didn't make a sound.

"Got it." Diana's latex gloves and the back of Cec's hand were spattered with blood. Diana wiped up what she could. She taped the IV needle into place and connected the tubes from the pouches to the back of the needle.

"You'll be more comfortable leaning back," she said to Cec and helped her adjust the pillows. "I'm giving you 2.5 milligrams. It should take effect in a few minutes. If that's not enough, let me know."

Cec nodded.

"A doctor will come by. I'm just not sure when."

I thought that Cec would eventually produce a Christmas present, but no gifts appeared in front of the wooden Christmas calendar. Mid-afternoon on Christmas Eve, Cec put on an apron and unwrapped the pork roast. We had both lived in Denmark and preferred a traditional Danish Christmas dinner. I hovered as she rubbed sea salt on the pork rind and asked what I could do to help. Nothing, I should just relax. I offered to peel the yams. No, she didn't need me underfoot. I should set the table and stay out of the way.

I watched as Cec mixed the marinade for the portobello mushrooms, shredded the Asiago. She cooked instinctively, understood food combinations, what paired well, how to season. She had an intuitive relationship with spices, would shake a small mound into her palm and consider, with a calculating squint, the exact requirement for a particular dish. Sometimes she'd come home with a flavour still in her mind and recreate a dish she couldn't forget. Or read through a recipe and understand how to torque it.

Like the lemon-blueberry pie from the little coffee shop in Benalto. None of the chairs or tables in the place matched. We sat hunched over our plates like weary cowhands and made small smacking noises of satisfaction. When the forks couldn't scrape up another crumb, we'd lifted our plates and licked.

"I'm going to have to make this," she'd said, and ordered a piece to go. "For further study."

Later at our dining table she chewed thoughtfully as she scribbled a list of ingredients, her guess at proportions. I sat across from her watching her fork travel from plate to mouth. Finally she put her pencil down and shoved the plate over to me. Two mouthfuls remained. "I can make this, and I can make it better."

Uh-oh, I thought, but I needn't have worried. She added extra lemon zest to heighten the sour sensation. This increased the sweet explosion of blueberry. A perfected pleasure.

She also tried a lemon-blueberry cheesecake on a graham wafer crust. The added richness was savour-worthy, but it was the pie I craved.

"I'm baking a lemon-blueberry," she'd say when I called to let her know I was on my way home from work. I'd press a little harder on the accelerator in an effort to get home before she'd wiped the flour dust from her cheek. If I reached her while she was still bent over sudsy dishwater, I'd wrap my arms around her from behind, my cheek against her cheek until I felt her jaw relax.

It was in those moments—the kitchen filled with warmth and comforting aromas, her generosity expansive—that made me want to keep coming home. I'd lived by myself for a long time. I liked opening the back door and stepping into the shared pleasure of home. I especially liked when she'd turn to me, her hands still wet with dishwater, her eyes smiling, and I'd kiss her falling-open mouth.

The brilliance of her Christmas dinner lay in her appreciation of a crispy but not overdone pork rind, the surprisingly fresh pop of new red potatoes smothered in a dark, salted Danish gravy that offset the mildly sweet yams.

"Cooking is all timing," she'd say to me, her jacket still on, just home from work on one of those days when she had worked late and I was making dinner. She'd lift the lid of a bubbling pot and say, "You started the pasta too soon." Or I'd chopped the carrots too fine, or let the broccoli steam too long.

The constant irritation in her voice—the growing certainty that nothing I did would ever be right—wore away at my confidence, my sense of capability. Her presence, or even her pending presence, could send me into a state of watchful apprehension.

Cec scored the pork rind so that when it baked it split into long, thin strips and was easy to break apart. The top was salty-crunchy and the underside fatty-soft. I held a strip between my thumb and forefinger and sucked at the fat. The rind broke apart between my teeth.

The squish of salty fat between my teeth reminded me of the cracklings my mother used to make. We'd eat them as a main course with freshly baked brown bread on which we'd spread the creamed honey from my grandfather, harvested from his industrious bees. On top of the honey we'd layer the cracklings, nubbly pork bits extracted from the fat that would congeal into lard. The cracklings were chewy and tasted salty. The sweet of the honey mashed together in my mouth with the fatty pork morsels and whole grain bread left my stomach warm and satisfied. Cec's Christmas dinner had the same effect.

I'd strung up Christmas lights in the living room and around the walls of our little dining area and Cec's work area. The whole house was an open area, more or less, with old walls at right angles that had settled into a crooked familiarity. No doors, except to the bathroom and the main floor bedroom. An arched opening connected the kitchen to the long stretch of living area. At one end of the living room, a couch and a love seat sat at right angles facing the TV. Behind the couch stood the table and chairs where we usually ate dinner, and at the far end, Cec's work area, an IKEA desk piled high, and a shelving unit stacked with books and papers.

We dimmed the lights, lit a candle, and said very little beyond "pass the gravy" and "this roast is tender."

Cec chewed slowly, watching me eat. She liked the way food made me happy. When I dished up seconds, she was still picking at her plate.

"Not hungry?"

She shrugged. "Not really."

"You've barely eaten anything."

This wasn't like her. I wondered at her lack of interest. When she quit smoking her greatest fear was that she would gain weight. Her solution? One meal a day. A firm rule. And she knew how to make that meal count. When we'd go to the Country Cousins in Linden for the dinner buffet—salad bar, borscht, home-baked buns, lemon chicken, handmade perogies, farmer sausage with bacon gravy, garden fresh peas—we'd both have the all-you-can-eat. She'd fill two plates, sometimes three.

One meal a day can't be good for her, I thought. But the small round of her tummy didn't get any bigger, or her hips. She didn't really have hips to speak of, no curves at all. She was slight and wiry. With her ball cap pulled low over her eyes she looked like an adolescent boy.

As I finished the last of my potatoes and gravy she sat staring at her plate, nudging the food with her fork but not actually eating.

"Are you done?" I asked as I picked up my plate. Cec had made the meal. The dishes were all mine.

After I'd finished the dishes, I found her on the couch in a dark, silent living room, leaning back, staring up at nothing. Her eyes rolled toward me as I handed her a present.

"We agreed. No presents."

"I know." But until that moment, I hadn't believed her. I set the present on her lap. It was larger than a coffee table book, and heavy.

"You really shouldn't have," she said, as she heaved her body upright into a sitting position, tilted her head down, and sent me a stern, reprimanding look over the rim of her glasses.

"It can be a gift for 'us,'" I offered, my cheeks getting hot.

She pulled the wrapping off *The Bobby Jones Collection*, a book and DVD set. More than once Cec had tuned in to watch old black-and-white films of Bobby Jones giving golf tips on the Golf Channel. She nodded when she saw Bobby's image on the front of the box. She lifted the lid to examine the contents. I was sitting on the love seat with Noddy curled up on my lap.

"Thank you." She set the box on the floor and leaned back again, closed her eyes.

Echo and Spidey, two of our eight cat, were curled on the chair behind Cec's desk. I thought I heard them purring, but maybe not. Maybe that was Stretch, who was on the prowl, stepping carefully along the back of the sofa. Cec had rescued her from the SPCA when she was a kitten. She was pitch black, part Persian, and generally cranky. She stepped from the back of the couch onto Cec's shoulder and then down her chest and onto her lap. Cec scratched her ear. "There's a good girl." Griff had clambered up onto the couch beside Cec. He wanted to lay his head in her lap but Stretch was there and he was wary.

"Lie down, Griff," Cec said, "lie down and be a good boy." He obliged, his head between his front paws. After a while he rolled over onto his side. By morning, he'd be asleep on his back, all four paws in the air.

Cec patted Stretch with long, firm strokes from her head all the way to her rump. Her purring grew louder and her front paws kneaded Cec's thighs while Cec sat staring at the silent TV. She was folded away into herself. I didn't have the faintest idea what she was thinking.

Sometimes I get a hit of her scent, the fresh mint of her shampoo, the deep woody waft of her skin, salt and earth laced with French lavender—that gangly herb with the teeny purple flowers that Cec had planted at the back of the herb bed.

She'd begun to wear her hair longer, gradually deepening the colour. No more short-cropped, bleached blonde. Because she was getting older, she said, her skin losing its luster. She teased her locks into curls with the blow dryer, wore flatter, more forgiving shoes. Fewer skirts and dresses. Earth tones. Lighter hues. No more dark-blue eye shadow (too thickly applied, I'd always thought).

A gust of leaves blows by, or a blonde in a leather coat swishes past me on the street, and Cec is instantly beside me, the top of her head level with my eyes, her bulging handbag bumping my thigh as we walk. I know it's her because of the way my chest tightens, my breathing slows. She is close enough to touch. If I could reach into that parallel dimension, I would kiss her. She wouldn't turn away.

"I like this place," Cec whispered, her eyes closed. The back of her bed was raised so that she was almost upright. For the first time in weeks the creases at the corners of her eyes were relaxed. "It's like someone has put a bit of happy in my veins."

I could barely make out "happy in my veins." Her jaw was slack. She was riding a morphine wave. The fluorescent bulb flickered above her head.

I sat with my head in my hands. I was so tired I could have curled up on the tile floor and fallen asleep. There was a relief in this place. Even though they couldn't tell us what was wrong. *Why hadn't she let me bring her in sooner?* I had been offering for weeks, trying to insist, ever since she'd said, "I think I have a health issue," on New Year's Day.

I closed my eyes, lulled by the murmur of nurses' voices, their soft-soled shuffle beyond the curtain.

I didn't realize it at the time but those were my hours of innocence. Cec's pain was under control, more or less, and I was still under the impression that pain could be controlled.

"Lyn?"

"Yeah?" I lifted my head.

"You need to call Lora."

"There are a few people I need to call."

"I don't want everyone to come." Cec's voice was suddenly stronger. "Not till we know what's going on."

I'd start with Lora, Cec's sister. And my mother. Mom would be concerned ("How is she?") and relieved ("I'm so glad she finally let you take her") with a hint of mild hysteria ("I hope it's nothing serious") and then crestfallen ("Oh…") when I'd tell her that she shouldn't come to the hospital.

Mom wouldn't push. She'd understand. Her relationship with Cec had never been easy. The first Christmas we were together, Mom had said that Cec wasn't welcome at our family Christmas dinner.

Not welcome? I had never heard this from my mother before. How many times had I eaten Christmas dinner with people I barely knew—a single mother from down the street with her young son, an elderly couple from church who didn't have any family close by, my brother's girlfriend du jour. My mother enjoyed feeding the hungry and she had a knack for rounding them up.

Her parents, my grandparents, were the same. When I was a kid and would spend a week at my grandparents' farm, there were usually a couple of teenage girls from the city there for the summer. Not foster kids exactly, but part of a program to keep disadvantaged youth off the streets, give them a positive experience of family. I'd grown up believing that hospitality was one of the fundamental tenets of the Mennonite faith, genetically encoded. "Not welcome" were words I'd never heard.

Cec said she understood, that she didn't take it personally. "Your mother loves you. She's being a mother hen. She thinks you need protection."

I told my mother that we would respect her wishes. Cec wouldn't come to Christmas dinner. But if Cec still wasn't welcome the next year, I wouldn't come either.

Mom didn't say anything, just looked at me with sad eyes. Ever since I'd come out to her, her face had sagged with a wounded sadness.

"Your mother's a drama queen," Cec said after our first dinner with my parents.

"This is difficult for her."

"Her tears are a manipulation."

"She thinks her daughter is going to hell."

"She really believes that?"

"She really does."

"I'm so sorry," Cec said, reaching for my hand.

"Sorry?" Cec almost never apologized. "For what?"

"For being in here. For putting you through this."

"No." I shook my head. "You don't have to apologize." But I understood why she felt the need to. She abhorred weakness, especially in herself, and would see her pain as an inexcusable shortcoming, a humiliation.

I took her hand. "This is where we need to be. I wouldn't want to be anywhere else."

"I was going to make us a special dinner tonight, for the Oscars."

Cec had written out a grocery list with instructions about where to go for each item. I'd put the list on the kitchen counter so I wouldn't forget. But then this morning she'd doubled over, grabbing onto the back of the sofa for support. When she looked up her face was white. "I can't do this anymore."

"They're finally giving you some worthwhile drugs." I attempted a smile.

"Drugs are good," she murmured. "When Diana comes I'm going to order another round."

"Is the pain back?"

"It never went away. But it's less."

A slender young woman in a white lab coat pulled back the curtain.

"I'm Dr. Somers." Her skin was pale, her dark shoulder-length hair perfectly straight and shiny, fingers long and bony. She seemed very young.

"Cecile Kaysoe?"

Cec and I both nodded.

Dr. Somers paused for a moment, consulted her clipboard, then looked up. "How's your pain?"

"Better, but not gone."

She flipped through the pages. "You're getting 2.5 mils. We could increase that to five, see if it helps."

"I don't want to be sleepy."

"The only way to find the right level is to try a little more and see what happens. If five makes you too sleepy, we can lower it next time."

Cec nodded. "Okay."

The young doctor set down her clipboard and asked Cec where her pain had started, when it had gotten worse, where she felt the pain most acutely, and whether it had been worse this morning. She lifted Cec's gown and pressed on Cec's abdomen. "How's this? And this? Have you been bloated? For how long?"

Cec's self-diagnosis: "Something in my female bits." In an email to one of her sisters Cec had written, "Worst case I'll have to have a hysterectomy. Not the end of the world."

Somers scribbled on her clipboard. "I'm going to order an X-ray and a CT scan. A GI specialist will come by to examine you. He's in surgery right now. I don't know how long he will be."

Cec pushed back the covers before light cracked the sky. From somewhere deep in the cave of sleep, my body felt a waft of cool air as she pushed herself upright. Did I hear the dull thud of her footsteps? The padding of dog paws toward the back door? She let the dogs out and set a pail under the kitchen tap to run water for the chickens, then a second pail. The sound of running water splashed through my mind. She pulled on her snow pants, her winter chore jacket, the rubber-soled barn boots with felt liners that came up to her knees.

The hinges croaked as she opened the back door. I lifted my head and squinted. I could see her out the bedroom window at the edge of the light, bundled against the cold, a bucket of water in each hand. Her boots crunched as she walked stiffly along the shoveled pathways watching to make sure the water didn't spill.

I let my head fall back onto the pillow. She didn't need to be up so early, not on New Year's Day, a morning specifically earmarked for sleeping in. But Cec's circadian rhythm didn't recognize weekends or holidays. She had no instinct for relaxation, no capacity for sleep beyond the minimum.

I had tried to explain the pleasure of sleeping in: as the brain begins to wake, the eyes remain closed and the body sinks into a weightless reverie, like floating, at the edge of consciousness. The body sleeps on while the brain watches and appreciates. It's an art form.

In Cec's world, the only real joy was physical labour: heaving, moving, digging, pounding, hauling.

I closed my eyes and rolled onto my side. I didn't want to get up.

But how could I stay in bed while she was out there in the freezing cold? I imagined pulling on my black one-piece chore suit, well insulated and heavy, with a canvas outer shell and hood. I could be out in -30°C with a raging wind and still be toasty. If the temperature climbed to -15°C or warmer, or if I moved a lot of bales, I'd end up drenched with sweat.

Usually Cec moved the bales, one at a time in a wheelbarrow, from the large stack beside the barn around to the other side of the small corral for the cows. She always fed the cows first, then the horses and llamas. If I went out with her, I'd feed the chickens, then the rabbits.

In order to step into that rhythm I needed to go out when she did. I'd already waited too long. By the time I got out the door she'd be on her way back in, or getting feed ready for the next round. If I offered to help, she'd wave me off. It was her workout, she said. No time to go to the gym so she got her exercise slinging fifty-pound bales, shoveling paths through the snow, heaving frozen cow patties into a big pile so the big, dumb cows wouldn't lie down in their own shit.

By the time she came in I was in the kitchen, my eyes squinting to adjust to the light as I tried in vain to pat down my bedhead of mouse-brown hair. I felt a blast of cold as the back door opened, then shut. She set the empty pails on the bench and bent to untie her boots. Mucus swung away from her nose and hung like a limp icicle. I handed her a tissue. She accepted without looking up. Her cheeks were red with cold, glasses fogged. Her head seemed small, swaddled in toque and scarves. Bundled up like that, her slight frame lost in the layers, she looked like a child—the same vulnerability that I felt in the sagging warmth of her bare skin when she wriggled closer in bed.

Over the last few days her silence had grown deeper. I knew better than to ask what she was thinking. But I also didn't want to just stand there like a lump.

I cleared my throat. "How is everyone?"

"Fine."

"Did you move bales?"

"No." She took four brown eggs from her jacket pocket and handed them to me. The eggs were still warm. She kept on her snow pants and didn't look at me as she walked past rubbing her hands together. The tepid warmth of our poorly insulated old farmhouse finally reached her and she shuddered. She sat down at her desk and flipped open her laptop but made no move to turn it on. She stared at the black laptop screen, then up at the television.

We'd had the television on almost continuously since the tsunami—the same clips over and over.

A cresting wave, rounded, and tall as a mountain, tumbled into froth, a thin frill on the horizon.

A grainy image wobbled, captured by a digital video camera held in an unpracticed tourist hand. A deep voice said, "*Was ist das?*" He zoomed in, then out. He panned to the shore and along a cement seawall that rose up ten feet above small, choppy waves. People were walking on the top of the wall behind a metal railing, looking out at the horizon and pointing.

The image shifted. A different video camera held by a steadier hand panning a different shoreline and a beach of white sand. Under the shade of a tree two young men were lounging in swim trunks on towels. One of them got up, his legs long and thin. He wrapped the towel around his waist and stood gesturing, saying something.

"That's Phuket, that beach," Cec said. "I've been there." She turned to me. "We should have been there."

She was right. We should have.

Cec's niece, Cassandra, almost twenty—precocious,

talkative, undecided about college, and restless—had decided to go back to Thailand where she had once spent a year as an exchange student. She had landed herself a paid position teaching English in Phuket and had assumed she could get a work permit when she got there.

"If Cass had gotten her permit before she left," I said, "we would have been there. On that beach. Today."

Cec would have been up early. I would have slept in. *Would Cec have known? When she saw the wave? Come running for me? Would we have made it to higher ground?* Or would we have ended up like Nate Berkus and his partner—one of them alive and the other pulled under, never to be found. I'd heard Nate's panicked voice on the radio. He couldn't find Fernando. That could have been us.

Cec got up and walked over to the patio door, opened it to let Echo in. He scurried inside then stopped, shook one paw at a time. She closed the patio door and stood staring out across the neighbour's snow-covered field. The wind whipped up miniature squalls that hurtled along, then subsided.

She'd gone quiet just before Christmas and had remained wrapped in a silence that grew deeper and wider with each day. When she wasn't doing chores she'd sit, often in front of her computer, staring. I wondered what thoughts were churning, and whether she was doing any writing? She had a way with words, and writing seemed to help her think. Occasionally she let me read what she'd written—pieces about her travels, or the farm.

I wished I had the courage to crouch down beside her, take her hand. But I didn't. I was almost certain she would respond with the sharp bite of recoil and I wasn't willing to put myself in the line of fire.

I thought about saying, "*Are you okay?*"

No, not that.

I wanted to ask, "*What are you thinking about?*"

I hesitated.

Because what if…

There were so many what ifs. *What if she was angry with me?*

I could hear her voice in my head: *The hutches need to be cleaned.*

Cec would say the garden needed weeding or the chickens needed to be cleaned out and I'd say that I would. But then I wouldn't.

"Why do you say that you'll do something if you have no intention…?"

I don't know—I was going to—

"Sometimes I think you are working out mother issues with me."

Mother issues?

"It's as though you need someone to resist."

I sank down onto the sofa, my head in my hands, staring at the TV. I was exhausted. Cec could go to bed at midnight or one in the morning and get up at five. Sometimes she didn't sleep at all, but that never slowed her down. My need for eight hours was incomprehensible to her. If I got ready for bed at ten, she'd look up from her computer and say, "It's still too early."

"I'll put in my ear plugs. You don't have to stop."

But already she'd be agitated.

I'd try to wait until eleven or twelve and end up falling asleep in front of the TV.

She'd nudge me. "You should have gone to bed!"

The only time I could sleep according to my body's natural rhythm without reprimand was when Cec was away on business.

"You like it when I leave," she'd say as she packed.

I'd deny, but she was right. When she was away, I could eat what I wanted to eat, sleep when I wanted to sleep, putter about the farm at a pace that worked for me.

I welcomed the solitude.

But living in this heavy silence, unbroken after so many days, was getting difficult to bear. The longer the silence stretched, the more inaccessible she seemed and the greater my sense of foreboding.

In all our time together, eight years and five months, I had never questioned, never wondered: if one of us was going to leave it would have to be me. It was one of the main reasons that I had kept making the decision to stay. She was the only person on the planet for whom I was the number one priority. If ever there was a major catastrophe, I'd be the one she'd think of first.

Now she was staring past me, tight-lipped. She'd gone quiet like this before. For days. Stone silent, even in bed.

I couldn't help wondering whether something had happened? *Could she tell that I'd been thinking about leaving?* It wouldn't surprise me. She was incredibly intuitive, moreso than I was comfortable with.

I hadn't said anything to her. I knew that if I ever said I was leaving, or that I was thinking about leaving, that would be it. She'd be done. Finished. I wasn't ready for that finality.

Whenever I thought about driving away for the last time, I'd see Noddy's happy little face, his trusting expectant eyes. I couldn't leave him behind. Cec would never let me take him.

Then there was the comfort of Cec's body curled up and gently snoring (when she did finally fall asleep) in bed beside me. I'd spent most of my life sleeping alone, eating alone, and knew how lonely a solitary existence could be. I wasn't in a hurry to go back to that.

When her mother began to decline, and Cec needed to take her to doctor's appointments, I had to keep the farm running, the animals fed. I couldn't walk away.

Then her mother died.

I stayed. But I made a decision: if Cec couldn't be

gentler, kinder, if we couldn't have fun, if her interest in sex didn't resurrect, I would leave. I would give her a year—to grieve her mother's death, to regain her equilibrium—but if nothing changed, I would go.

Her mother had died in April, nine and a half months ago. Only two and a half months left.

I didn't tell Cec about my plan. She'd say I was being manipulative. Or she'd say I didn't love her, never had.

I made toast for lunch, with tuna and tomato and ate by myself. I set my plate in the sink beside the bowl from breakfast and my mug with tea remains. Cec was at her desk, computer on. Noddy was lying belly-up on her lap and she was rubbing his tummy, absently. She barely glanced in my direction.

I could say something that would irritate her, provoke annoyance, but I didn't have the energy.

I sat on the couch, my back to her. Stretch jumped up onto my lap. Griffy laid his big head on my knee. I wanted to be anywhere but sitting here watching the snow swirl, filling the tire tracks on the driveway, living in this perpetuation of absence—at a growing distance from my friends, living in a poorly insulated farmhouse out in the middle of empty prairie.

I listened for the scrape of Cec's chair, her steps across the floor. Even if she said nothing, I expected her to give me an appraising look over the top rim of her glasses: *What are you doing? Just sitting there?*

Nothing.

I heard her pour hot water into a mug, swish the tea bag.

I had let this happen—this apprehensive silence, this disconnect from my former life.

When I called my mom, or anyone, Cec was always there, always enquiring. No conversation belonged to just me anymore.

I imagined Cec bringing the mug to her lips, blowing gently, one arm folded across her middle.

Maybe my worry was misplaced. When her mother died, Cec had taken a few days off, helped arrange the funeral. She'd been her usual calm, capable self, but sad-eyed, pensive. Two days after her mother's memorial, she went back to work. Maybe this silence was her grief, delayed.

Or maybe she was sick. I'd seen her grimace and bend, holding her stomach. When I asked her what was wrong, she waved me away. "Just a cramp."

I suggested she see the doctor.

"Had my fill of doctors when my mother was sick."

I had too. Her mother's demise had consumed the bulk of two years with doctor's appointments, prescriptions, hospitalizations, long-term care.

Toward the end, the nursing home had moved Cec's mother out of her shared room and into a very small private room, just large enough for a bed and two chairs. When I arrived that final evening, the air was sour with the smell of illness. Cec's mother's eyeballs were bulging behind closed lids, her lungs sucking hard for air through dry lips. I was surprised how ashen her skin looked, how sunken her cheeks were.

Cec took her mother's hand and squeezed as she leaned in close.

"Mom, it's Lyn. Lyn's here. She's come to see you."

She struggled to open her eyes and tried to focus. Her eyes met mine and I could see she was still there, dim but comprehending, unable to form words. I stood shoulder to shoulder with Cec, my eyes watering, nauseated by the smell.

That was the last time Cec's mother opened her eyes. The nurses said that her brain died first, from lack of oxygen. Lungs and heart are often the last to give in, stubbornly refusing to give up their instinctive rhythm. Cec said that her mother was mad; she didn't want to die.

A crust formed on her lips and her mouth took on an even more pronounced *0* shape, like a goldfish.

It was the middle of the night. I was tired. My willingness to hold vigil had been worn down by the hours. The nurse was giving her enough morphine to slow her breathing but not enough to kill her. With each exhale we wondered whether—and I hoped that—it would be her last.

The rest of the family left, one by one. Somehow these final hours were allotted to Cec, and Cec was loath to leave. But she had the strong sense that her mother didn't want her to stay, and her mother, Cec knew, was many times more stubborn than any of her children.

Eventually Cec beckoned and I followed. She stopped at the front desk and asked the nurse to be sure someone called her if…when…

She said nothing as she drove to our hotel. She had checked us into a hotel so we could be close by. Noddy was waiting for us there, curled up on the bed.

I don't think Cec slept.

Her cell rang at 5:12 a.m.

"Okay," she said.

I switched on the bedside light.

"Uh-huh. When did she go? Oh. Okay. Thank you." She flipped her cellphone shut, pulled the blankets up to her chin. "Turn that off," she said.

"When did she go?"

"She was pronounced around 5 a.m. but I don't think they know exactly."

Cec lay staring at the ceiling. I rolled onto my side.

"If they ask," Cec said, "we were there when she went."

I didn't say anything.

"I said we'd stay," she said.

"She was pretty much gone when we left."

"She didn't want us there."

"No, she didn't."

I lay with my eyes open, Noddy stretching beside me. Soon he would tiptoe between our bodies up to our faces then collapse onto one of our pillows.

That morning it was my face he smothered with his curly fur. If I didn't move, he'd go back to sleep. I lay there listening to the rattle of his small exhales. They sounded almost like a purr. The rattle in his lungs was the only remaining sign that he had been driven over by the back tire of a neighbour's half-ton. Somehow he'd survived.

Cec got up. She didn't turn on any lights, went into the bathroom, and closed the door. The toilet flushed. When she came out, she pulled on her turtleneck, jeans, pullover, jacket, toque, mitts. Noddy had already bounced off the bed and was circling her ankles. I heard the click of his leash. The door opened to a flood of hallway light, then a sigh of air as she eased the door closed behind her.

What would she have done if she'd come home after work one day and I was gone?

I imagined her setting down her briefcase, slowly, when she saw the empty bookshelves and then the realization beginning to sink in. She would find my note and stand reading, arms crossed, her face expressionless.

If I ever came home to a closet emptied of her clothes, I would sit and stare out the window. But Cec's remedy for everything was hard physical labour. Sweat it out. She would put on her chore coveralls and head outside to feed the animals, muck out the corrals.

If Cec ever decided to leave, she would do it when I was gone. She wouldn't belabour the details or stick around for the fallout. Once she made a decision, that was that.

When we crawled into bed that night I tried to make my breathing sound like I was drifting off. I knew I wasn't fooling her. She wasn't sleeping either.

"What is it?!" she said finally. The sound of her voice came as a surprise; it was the first time she'd asked me a direct question in days. I didn't answer. I turned away. If I said anything she would hear the quaver in my voice.

"Oh, come on! What's going on?"

I swallowed and tried for a steady voice. "Something's wrong. I don't know what."

She took a deep breath. "It's not always about you, you know."

I rolled toward her. "Then what is it?"

She was silent.

I waited.

"I've known this for a while." We were lying on our backs. My face was turned to her. She was staring at the ceiling. "I probably should have done something about it sooner."

I waited.

"I have a serious health issue…"

A serious health issue? My heart was pounding in my ears.

"…but I don't want to talk about it."

How serious?

"Okay," I said, slowly letting out my lungful of air. "You don't have to talk about it. But can you tell me what it is?"

Movement under the covers. Her fingers touched the inside of my forearm and slid down along my arm. "I don't know." She took my hand. "I have a pain in my stomach. That's all I know."

I couldn't sleep. I lay wide-eyed, staring at the ceiling. *She'd known—the pain—she hadn't said anything—again—*

shut me out. That's where I lived—always—on the outside of her inner conversation.

I tried to squeeze back my tears.

She hated it when I cried: "Your tears are manipulative."

I'd turn away but I wasn't always fast enough and she could usually tell anyway.

After what Cec had admitted the night before about the pain in her abdomen I thought she might finally be ready to talk. But no, she offered nothing all day.

I wanted to ask her when she'd first noticed, but I held my tongue. I was worried, and also mad—a jaw-grinding anger—that she hadn't said anything, just closed up and left me to think her silence was about me, again. If we hadn't talked last night would she have kept her pain to herself? Gone off to the doctor without telling me?

After dinner Cec called the dogs then looked at me and nodded toward the door. I got my jacket. The sky was moonless, pitch black. Griff charged ahead, Noddy and Charlie running hard after him. As soon as the dogs left the ring of porch light, they were swallowed by darkness. I could hear the crunch of their paws on the snow.

The cold air stung my cheeks. The sky was so black I couldn't see the ground, couldn't even see Cec's face. I wanted to be able to see the dogs. I wished Cec would take my hand.

One of the dogs brushed against my leg. I slowed my steps as I heard a small yip. *Noddy?* I didn't like not being able to see him. *What if there was a coyote?*

Cec stopped. "Let's head back." She whistled and the dogs stampeded past us back down the driveway. I matched my stride to hers.

"I'm going to a clinic in the morning," she said. "A walk-in. It'll be faster."

About bloody time! I thought but didn't say it.

"I don't want you to say anything to anyone."

Not even my mother? I had wanted to call Mom all day but hadn't. I knew what Cec would say. *This is personal. It isn't anyone's business.*

"Okay, I won't. Until we know."

Cec wouldn't let me drive her to the clinic. "You can't miss work, Lyn, that makes no sense!"

So we left the next morning like we always did. Me first, out into the cold and dark of an early winter morning, onto a road covered with snow, headlights illuminating the white flashes of flakes.

I should have been more insistent about taking her to the clinic. *Would it have made a difference?*

The snow was falling heavily, the pavement covered. I inched along, straining to make out the downward slope of the ditch.

The previous winter, I'd been driving this same stretch of road through blowing snow. I'd felt the slide of ice under my tires as I drove up the hill by Hank and Doreen's. There was a glow of headlights coming toward me from the other side. Snow covered the dividing line. I wanted to be sure I was far enough over so I'd turned the steering wheel, just barely, and felt my back end swing. I lifted my foot from the accelerator and tried to keep the wheels straight. I didn't want to swerve into the oncoming vehicle.

We crested the hill at the same time. A white half-ton. As I passed him, I felt my wheels skid. I tapped the brake. Sheer ice. My back end swung out and I couldn't straighten. I turned toward the ditch. Better to hit the ditch here where it was shallower than farther along where the incline was steep. I hurtled down, then up, missing a telephone pole by a foot, slamming sideways into, and through, a barbed-wire fence. The vehicle remained upright, skidding down the slope of the pasture.

When I jolted to a stop, the engine was still running, my foot solidly jammed on the brake, my heart pounding. I turned off the ignition. Cec would say I'd been driving too fast. *But I wasn't!* I could already hear myself insisting.

I pulled out my cell. No reception. I opened the car door and sank down into snow past my knees.

The half-ton had turned around—he'd seen me fishtail. He lived just a mile up the road and was driving his son to school. Was I okay? Did I need a ride?

I was relieved that I hadn't hit him. My eyes filled with tears as his son slid over on the seat. He was holding tight to his lunch pail with both hands. The warmth of the truck was reassuring. I was shaking.

Cec met me at the back door.

"Car's in the ditch," I said in a whisper. I could barely get the words out.

Her hand flew to her chest. She fell back half a step, her eyes wide. I'd never seen this look on her face before, a raw terror at the thought of losing me. I felt a swell of reassurance in that moment; if something happened to me it would matter to her.

"I'm okay," I said, reaching for her. She was trembling. "I'm right here," I took her hand and squeezed it. "I'm okay. Missed the hydro pole."

"Where—"

"Hank and Doreen's pasture."

She squeezed my hand, a vice grip. "I don't know what I'd do…" Then gathered herself. "Don't do this to me! I couldn't bear it."

My cellphone vibrated.

"Got here in one piece." Cec sounded relieved. I was too. The drive into Calgary from the farm took about an hour if road conditions were good, longer on snow and ice.

"This waiting room is full. Could be a while."

"You knew it would be."

She lowered her voice. "The mix of people in here is interesting. Everyone from junkies to lawyers."

"Any junkie lawyers?"

I could hear her smile. "I'm in good company."

She'd driven all the way downtown to Eighth and Eighth. There were clinics that were closer, but Cec's natural inclination would be the hubbub of downtown, the odd mix of humanity. With her black ball cap pulled down over her eyes, she'd sit slouched in a waiting room chair and observe.

I left Cec's cubicle and walked down the Emergency hallway past half-pulled curtains. I heard a small child crying in gasps. A man lay on a stretcher in a neck brace, blood on his face. Two blue-uniformed paramedics stood over him, each with a protective hand on the stretcher rail. The wide glass Emergency room doors slid aside automatically.

There was a NO CELLPHONES sign in the waiting room so I walked over to the pay phone and dug around in my pocket for thirty-five cents. I dialed Lora's number, Cec's youngest sister. She was three years older than me and seven inches shorter.

Lora said she would come right away. And no, she wouldn't call anyone else, not even Dennis and Nell, Cec's brother and sister-in-law.

"Not until we know what's going on." I could hear myself parroting Cec.

Next I called Doreen. She was surprised. "In the hospital? What happened?"

"Pain in her abdomen."

"She never said—"

"She didn't want anyone to know."

"I hadn't heard from her in a while. I thought she was away."

"She went into Emergency in Three Hills. And also Didsbury."

"What did they say?"

I hesitated. Doreen had been a nurse before she'd retired to help Hank on the farm. She would understand, better than most, but that was also part of the problem. I could hear Cec's voice: *Don't tell everyone.* Cec had said little to anyone. The doctor at the clinic had sent her for an ultrasound. The results showed a two-inch mass on her right ovary. She was referred to a gynecologist. The gynecologist recommended surgery to remove the mass.

I wanted to tell Doreen about the mass, the escalation of her pain, the surgery. I wanted to ask Doreen what questions I should be asking, how worried I should be.

"The X-rays show some osteoarthritis in her back," I said, which was true. "But her pain kept getting worse. This morning she couldn't stand it anymore."

Dorothy didn't say anything for a moment. Then: "You need us to do chores?" Ever the pragmatist.

"If you could, please. I'll try to get home tonight, but I'm not sure how late."

When I got back to Cec's curtained cubicle, Dr. Somers was at her bedside again. I heard the word "ultrasound."

"They did one when I went to the clinic," Cec said.

"We need to do another one. They can bring a portable unit."

The first time I met Doreen, she drove into our yard on a warm fall afternoon, didn't bother with calling. At the time we were still new to the farm and to the country custom of driving onto a farmyard unannounced.

By the time I opened the back door, Doreen was striding toward the house. She was wearing a short-sleeved, plaid shirt, her hair grey and curly.

"I'm Doreen Loewen," she said, her voice surprisingly raspy. "My husband, Hank, combined your field, that bit up there."

She was sizing me up, her eyes missing nothing. I knew that Cec had made an arrangement through one of the neighbours to have someone swath and bale the section of pasture we called "the small triangle," an extension of the top pasture. I'd seen someone on a swather one day, and a week later when we got home from work there were neat stacks of bales, ten to a pile, dotting the small patch of pasture.

"We haven't been paid," Doreen said.

"Oh. Sorry. How much?"

"Fifty dollars, plus tax."

"I don't think I have enough cash. Cheque okay?"

She nodded.

When I came out again Doreen was scanning the yard. "You like it out here?"

I nodded.

"Move from the city?"

"Yeah."

"Just the two of you?"

It was clear that she knew the answer. "Yes," I said, "just the two of us." So far her questions hadn't felt invasive.

"Fred and Linda made some nice improvements to the place." She gestured in the direction of the corrals.

"Yes, they did." They had torn down the old corral and built two new ones, a large one on the north side of the barn and a smaller one on the south side. Fred had cemented the posts into the ground and attached the corral boards with bolts. Cec thought it was overkill.

"They didn't move very far—"

"No, they didn't." They had bought a fixer-upper a mile down the road.

"I thought they'd move to town," Doreen said. "Fred's away so much."

"Yemen." I nodded, smiling at my first contribution to farmer-gossip. I handed Doreen the cheque. "Thank you."

"We're just up the road if you need anything."

"We're here to do an ultrasound?" A young woman was pulling a monitor on a stand. A young man pushed from behind. They both wore white lab coats. The sum total of their ages probably didn't add up to Cec's. I wondered how they had managed to find themselves rolling an ultrasound machine around an Emergency Ward. Was this a conscious choice? Always wanted to work in radiology? Or was this accidental?

That's what had happened to me—an accidental career. After university, I'd landed a job as a proposals manager at Hanson Consoles, a small, family-owned millwork shop that had been making high-end boardroom tables, bookshelves, credenzas, and map drawers for the oil companies in downtown Calgary for thirty years. Despite the rollercoaster of an oil and gas economy, the business had grown to fill a thirty-thousand-square-foot manufacturing facility. When Tom took over the business from his dad he'd wanted a more stable revenue stream and began building consoles—specialized furniture with a steel frame structure designed to withstand the 24/7 demands of computer-intensive control-room environments. Within a year I had been promoted from proposals to sales.

I'd never imagined myself in sales, probably because my father was a salesman. He'd begun his working life as a highschool history teacher, then sold World Book Encyclopedia during the summer to make extra money. Soon he was making more selling encyclopedias than he would ever make teaching.

When he was home for dinner, which wasn't often, the teacher in him couldn't resist a captive audience. I'd sat through many sales seminars at the dinner table, learned all about "qualifying questions" and the "soft close." I had never imagined that I would one day discover I had a natural aptitude for sales. Neither did my father. He called me an "artsy-fartsy." We both thought I'd end up living in an attic or a one-room studio subsisting on the returns of my creative endeavours.

The young woman smeared a clear jelly across Cec's belly and pressed the blunt end of a wand against her skin. Almost instantly a grainy black-and-white image appeared on the computer screen.

The young man frowned. "Have you had something to eat recently?"

Cec shook her head, then remembered, "Oh, egg salad sandwich."

"When was that?"

"An hour ago?"

"That would do it. We won't be able to get a clear image until that egg salad has cleared the digestive tract."

Lora was waiting for me in the Emergency waiting room, her eyes watery. "She must be in a lot of pain to let you bring her here."

"She's at the end of the hall." I nudged Lora forward.

Cec's eyes fluttered open when I pulled back the curtain that surrounded her stall. She squinted and shielded her eyes with her hand.

"Hey, old girl." Lora tried to smile but her voice wavered. "What are you doing in here?"

"Hey you," Cec said in a dry-mouth whisper. She motioned Lora closer.

Lora squeezed Cec's hand and kissed her cheek. I rolled a stool closer so she could sit.

"Lyn says they're giving you good drugs."

"They are, finally. And no, I'm not sharing."

I left to check on Noddy and put money in the meter. When I came back, Cec was gone. A porter had come to take her down for a CT scan. Lora was rummaging in her handbag for a cigarette.

"Where do I go?" she asked, holding it up.

I walked down the hall with her, through the waiting

room, out the Emergency doors, down the sidewalk. The sunshine was glaring, the wind brisk. Lora had trouble getting her cigarette lit. I stood close to shield her flickering flame. Her hand trembled as she took a drag and held it to ensure the nicotine reached all her nerve endings.

"She's a stubborn shit." Lora gave an uneasy laugh as she exhaled.

"With the highest pain threshold of anyone I've met."

"Why the hell can't someone figure out what's wrong with her?"

"At least they're taking her pain seriously."

"She says you're like a hovering grandmother."

"I try not to."

"She can't stand needing help. Gets that from my dad."

"Your mother wasn't exactly a pushover either."

"That's true. Especially when she lost her marbles. She got so stubborn about stupid stuff. But you know that. You saw her a lot near the end."

I nodded. "The more I got to know your mother, the more Cec made sense."

"Oh god, don't tell her that!" Lora looked like she was about to laugh, and cry.

"She comes by her bullheadedness honestly."

Lora grinned. "I'll never forget the day she called to tell me about you."

Cec had been in the kitchen putting away clean dishes. I was in the living room and could hear Cec's end of the conversation.

"We had friends over, playing cards," Lora said. "I'd had a few beer."

Cec said later she should have known better. She could tell Lora was drunk, or at least well lubricated. But she had already told Dennis and she didn't want Lora to hear it from someone else.

"Cec said that she was seeing someone. I thought that

was weird because I already knew she was seeing someone. What was that guy's name?"

"Andy."

"The tennis player—"

"Yeah."

I'd heard Cec say, "A woman, Lora…No, I'm not kidding!"

"Took a minute to sink in," Lora said. "I wasn't expecting anything like that. I hadn't ever wondered. And then it hit me—my sister's a lezzie!"

"Cec said you yelled it."

"I didn't yell—did I?"

Cec had held the phone away from her ear. "Lo—Lora, keep it down. The whole world doesn't need to know!"

A bearded doctor in green scrubs pulled back the pastel curtain that surrounded Cec's Emergency Ward bed. He had bushy eyebrows and what looked like a light-green shower cap on his head.

He pressed Cec's abdomen. He asked her to recount her symptoms for him, the escalation of her pain.

The pain had started in her abdomen then moved to her back.

None of the doctors she'd seen had seemed overly concerned—not her family doctor, not the doctor at the Three Hills Emergency Ward when her pain suddenly got worse, or the doctor she went to see in Didsbury when she became desperate for a stronger painkiller.

Cec grimaced when the surgeon in the green scrubs pressed down on her stomach. He asked how frequently she had to pee and whether she had any difficulty with bowel movements.

Cec had always had a problem with her bowel movements. Chronic constipation. She was constantly experimenting with herbal supplements. Her current favorite was Stomach Ease.

She listed her remedies for him:

Cayenne pepper, for circulation
Calcium, for her bones
Magnesium, to aid in the absorption of calcium
Chlorophyll, for fresh breath
Gingko Biloba, for energy
Ginseng, for digestion
Vitamins C, D, E

I should have asked what they were they testing for. I didn't. I stood with my hands shoved into my jeans. Cec didn't ask either.

Interesting how docile we both became, willing to be handled. It made no sense, this compliant silence from two intelligent professionals who understood the utility of a well-formulated question. Neither of us asked.

As soon as the doctor was gone, an attendant appeared with a wheelchair to take Cec down for an X-ray.

I stood beside Cec's empty hospital bed feeling unwashed and lumpy, wishing I'd taken a shower. Cec had been packed and ready to go when I'd come in from chores and I hadn't wanted to give her an opportunity to change her mind. I'd pulled on a baseball cap, a golf shirt and fleece. Didn't bother to look in the mirror. I knew what I'd see: tummy bulging over waistband, cheeks covered in tiny suffering welts.

"You're eating chocolate again." Cec would take my chin between her thumb and forefinger and turn my face side to side scrutinizing the pimples clustered in patches on my cheeks. "You shouldn't pick your face."

"I don't pick," I said, as I lifted her fingers from my face. "I tweeze."

The truth was that in between tweezing stray hairs from my chin, I would squeeze (or attempt to squeeze) the hardened kernel out of a blackhead or the puss out of a zit.

Were the stray hairs on my chin a sign of too much testosterone in my bloodstream? Was it a hormonal imbalance that had drawn me to Cec?

I sank down into the chair beside her empty bed and leaned my head against the cinder block wall. I should call Tom, my boss. I'd thought about it when I was at the pay phone. But what reason could I give for not coming into work when all I was doing was sitting uncomfortably in a hospital room staring at the wall?

What I knew for sure was that I didn't want to leave this

room. I wanted to be here when Cec got back.

I stretched out my legs and shifted from one bum cheek to the other. My eyes closed, lulled by the rumble of gurney wheels on the other side of the curtain, the rise and fall of voices. I thought about the emails waiting for me at work, and the voicemails, clients expecting price quotes and layout drawings.

The doctor in the green scrubs returned. He didn't turn on the light and stood for a moment with one arm folded across his middle.

"I'm sorry we have to keep disturbing you." He stroked the bristles on his chin. "I wish I could tell you that I know conclusively what we're dealing with. Unfortunately, all I can tell you is that we need to run more tests." He paused. "Getting the tests done will be easiest if we admit you as a patient. We'll be able to fit you in more easily when there's an opening."

"That's fine," Cec said, glancing at me as she suppressed a smile. None of the doctors she'd seen had seemed overly concerned about her pain and she was happy someone was finally taking her seriously.

"I'm sorry," he said, "I know this has been a long day."

Cec waved away his apology. "Really. It's okay."

"You'll have to make arrangements. I don't know exactly how long. You should probably plan to be here for three or four days. As soon as there's a bed available, they'll move you up."

After he left, Cec pumped her fist, "Yes!" with a triumphant smile.

I'd been gathering myself to stand firm, insist that they admit her. I tried to smile.

"Oh, don't cry, Lyn! Not in here. You know how I hate tears.

Cec had been so irritatingly stubborn about not letting me drive her to her doctor's appointments. I'd insisted. She'd resisted. I could see the determination in her eyes. She wasn't about to lean on anyone, least of all me.

When her gynecologist suggested surgery to remove the lump, Cec seemed satisfied. Surgery would resolve her issue. She hadn't counted on the pain getting worse: "Sharper. Like a knife in my back."

"Let me take you in to Emergency in Calgary."

"No!" She kept going to see small-town doctors. During one of her visits to a doctor in Didsbury he'd said, in a kindly tone, "We all have a few aches and pains as we get older." She didn't tell me this until later, and it was obvious by her tone that she had heard his words as a kind of empathy. "A few aches and pains!" I was incensed.

"Settle down." She waved away my agitation. "It's not that big a deal."

I wondered exactly how long the Didsbury doctor would be able to bear up under the "aches and pains" Cec was dealing with minute by minute, hour by hour.

She stopped going into the office, working as much as she could from home, often standing at her laptop, sometimes pacing. When she couldn't stand the pain, she'd go outside, grab the pitchfork, and heave cowpies.

"Did you move bales?" I asked one evening when she came in from chores.

She sank onto the bench in the back entrance and bent over to take off her boots. "Not all of them."

"Do you want me to move the rest?"

"Do I have to spell it out?!"

"I'm sorry. I thought—" I'd been working so hard not to worry, not to hover.

"Don't apologize!"

"You don't want me to apologize, or worry, or drive you anywhere. What exactly do you want me to do?"

She pulled off her jacket, moving slowly. "You'll have to do the outside for a while. I'll do the house."

That she didn't have the strength to sling bales was a huge admission.

I took over feeding the animals. She washed dishes, swept the floor. I did the vacuuming.

She asked me to bring home tins of paint, a medium blue and a darker blue, which she used to paint the legs of our IKEA dining table and the backs and legs of the chairs. She painted the closet doors of the two freestanding closets, the one in the bedroom and the one in her work area. Everything blue. She said the movement of the paintbrush took her mind off the pain.

And she could still cook. I'd arrive home from work to veggies steaming, meatloaf bubbling, muffins just out of the oven, an experimental sweet potato pie that could be eaten as dessert or served as a side.

I didn't have an appetite but I forced myself to chew. I was having a hard time concentrating at work. I rushed home, pushing the speed limit, afraid that I'd find her collapsed on the kitchen floor.

I fully expected that one day the pain would become more than she could stand and I was afraid of what might happen. Best case would be an empty house and a note from Doreen. Cec wouldn't call 911 but she might call Doreen.

Another appointment with the gynecologist. For the first time Cec didn't fight me when I offered to drive. But only to the front door. No, I couldn't come in.

I watched, helpless, as she walked slowly through the sliding doors. She was tough as a bed of nails I told myself. She would find a way to wriggle out from under. But no matter how firmly I talked to myself, I couldn't escape the increasingly obvious. She was slipping, sliding.

I went to work but couldn't concentrate. All morning I felt nauseated. At noon my cellphone finally buzzed.

"Hurt like hell." Cec's voice sounded strained and very far away. Then, in an even smaller voice, she said, "I'm bleeding pretty heavily."

"I'm coming."

She didn't object. She didn't say that she was fine and I shouldn't worry. She just said, "I'm at the Chapters across the street."

I accelerated through yellow lights. *What had he done to her?* I forced myself to walk, not run, through the front doors. *Where was she?* I pulled out my cell to dial her number and caught sight of her, standing beside the wall of books that lined the back of the store. She waited until I reached her.

"Hey!" I tried to sound nonchalant but I was breathless. She looked china doll fragile. I was careful not to touch her.

"Did you find what you were looking for?"

She shook her head. "But I found this." She held up *Traveling Mercies* by Anne Lamott. "Remember *Bird by Bird?*"

Yes, I remembered *Bird by Bird*. Cec had read it. A book on writing. She'd suggested I read it. I'd never finished.

Cec said she wanted to look at the magazines. She motioned with her chin toward the racks at the other end of the store. I didn't offer my arm. She objected to physical contact in public. I walked slowly, stayed close. After several shuffling steps, I felt her hand on my elbow. I was surprised. She had never taken my arm in public before. We proceeded slowly, as though she were eighty years old and I were her daughter.

"Just put all her stuff on the bed," Diana said. "We'll roll her right into her new room."

"I don't even have to get out of bed?"

"You can lie there like a princess."

I picked up Cec's purse.

"No, give me that, I'll hold it."

I tossed Cec's jacket onto the foot of her bed, along with my jacket, her slippers, bottles of water, and my backpack.

"You'd think we'd taken up permanent residence!" Cec frowned as she watched the pile on the bed grow.

"Ready?" Diana shoved the curtain aside and flipped up the brakes on the bed. Two male porters appeared. They manoeuvred the bed while Diana, Lora, and I followed behind.

When our procession arrived at the entrance to Ward 51, we waited while Diana conferred with a nurse at the nurses' station. When she returned she directed us to roll Cec's bed backward, to a room immediately left of the main doors. Room #1. The porters eased the bed around the tight corner and positioned Cec under a flickering fluorescent bulb. A curtain divided the room in half. On the other side we could see the wheels of another bed.

"Mmm, a roommate." Cec's brow furrowed. "Well at least there's a bathroom. Put my purse in that." Cec pointed at a narrow locker. "And hang my clothes. I need a bottle of water on this table where I can reach it. And my books."

There was room for a row of visitors' chairs at the foot of the bed and space for one person to pull up a chair on either side.

Lora hung back in the doorway. "I'll take Noddy," she said in a small voice.

"That would be great, Lora." I wanted to take Noddy home to the farm with me but tomorrow would be another long hospital day and I didn't want him to spend it locked in a vehicle.

Cec dictated the list of supplies I should bring from the farm: underwear, newspaper, her old glasses, and the books from her bedside table, Tom Harpur's *The Pagan Christ* and John Grisham's *The Broker*.

"I thought you already read the Grisham."

"Not quite finished."

Cec had all of Grisham's books in softcover, all of Ludlum, and pretty much all of a murder series where each book is a letter: *K is for Killer*. I didn't know the author. Didn't care.

Cec had always objected to my books—the space they took up, the number of hardcovers; they were too expensive and too unwieldy to fit in a carry-on. She rolled her eyes at my Urquhart, Munro, Shields, Engel.

"Pretentious," Cec had said of Atwood. "Canadian writers take themselves so seriously."

"Don't forget the Russians." I handed her Dostoyevsky, Akhmatova, Nabokov. "Or the Czechs." Škvorecký. "And the Poles." Miłosz.

"Have you read *The Bourne Identity*?"

I shook my head.

"I think you'd like it."

I doubted that I would. But on my next business trip I found a well-thumbed copy of *The Bourne Identity* in my suitcase.

I hadn't seen Cec pick up a book in weeks—pain had diminished her ability to focus—but I could understand her desire to have them on her bedside table.

"Could you get me my purse?" Cec asked as I put on my jacket.

I retrieved her purse from the locker. She pulled out her wallet and handed me her cash, about a hundred dollars, then decided to keep twenty dollars: "Just in case." She gave me her credit cards: "Not safe in a place like this."

I also had instructions to take dog food over to Lora's, buy a flat of Co-op Gold water, pick up a paper and some apples. McIntosh.

The prairie rolled and heaved, dimly illuminated by the moon. I could see all the way to the horizon—a ghostly plain. I was driving toward a single, naked yard light. The house would be cold and empty.

I lifted my foot from the accelerator. I wanted to go home to the farm. And I wanted to be with Cec. I didn't like the idea of her being alone when she was in pain—and vulnerable. I let the car glide. *Should I? Where would I sleep? In one of those rigidly uncomfortable chairs?* No, she wouldn't want me there. And I needed to check on Griff and Charlie.

What I really, really wanted was to be heading home knowing that Cec would be in full swing with spring cleanup, garden prep, building projects. I never knew exactly what idea was taking shape in her head when she emerged from the barn with the Skil saw in her hand, a yellow extension cord over her shoulder. She'd set the saw on the long workbench beside the small corral and go back to the barn for her toolbox, ratchet set, power drill, and hammer, a pencil tucked behind her ear.

"What are you building?" I'd ask. Couldn't help myself even though I knew she probably wouldn't tell me.

"A surprise," she'd say, as she headed back toward the barn.

"If you're going to countersink, this must be serious."

I picked up my pitchfork and went into the small corral. As I scooped cow patties and heaved them onto a growing pile, I could hear her sawing, hammering, drilling, then more hammering.

I was almost finished pitching chicken shit and straw into the wheelbarrow when Cec called, "Come have a look!"

She was standing beside a finished cage. Three of the sides were covered in mesh with plywood on the floor, back, and top. The top had a round hole cut in it and on the front there was a door that took up the middle third. The cage was about two-and-a-half-feet wide, a foot-and-a-half deep, and about a foot-and-a-half high.

"A nursery!" I said.

She nodded, grinning. "And see, I cut out a hole on top so we can mount a heat lamp."

"The baby chicks are going to love you for this!"

"A new condo with room service."

"I love you for it too," I said, and stepped closer to kiss her.

Cecile Georgina Burdett was born to Patricia (nee McLaren) Burdett and Jim Burdett on May 5, 1952, in Calgary, Alberta, Canada.

She came into the world with a shock of black hair and olive skin. Cec told me that her father called her "Little Eskimo." "Are you sure she's mine?" he asked, holding her up. Her father's lips were smiling but his eyes appraising as he watched his wife for any sign of guilt.

For a full year, Cecile was doted on by a mother who loved newborns, enjoyed nursing, felt relaxed and contented with the weight of an infant wriggling against her shoulder. But as Cec began to fill out, her mother's belly began to grow too. The space on her mother's lap shrank away until there was barely room for a tottering infant reaching up to be held. Eventually, her mother's lap disappeared completely. The Little Eskimo watched. She understood.

One of Cecile's older sisters said she remembers Cec, as a toddler, watching her with a solemn gaze, as though she could discern the truth. She was the middle child. Number six of eleven. Five brothers. Five sisters. For several years she shared a bed with two of her sisters. One of the sisters was a bed-wetter. I can't remember who it was and it doesn't matter, the point being that sharing a bed was more damp and unpleasant than comfortingly communal.

I know that her family moved, more than once. For a number of years they lived in a house on Stanley Road in Calgary that overlooked the Stampede Grounds. I don't know how old Cec was when they lived there.

She also told me about a farm without plumbing or heating that was brutally cold in the winter. They only lived there a year, too hard to keep children bathed without running water.

There was another farm too, at what is now the intersection of Shaganappi and Crowchild Trail. Cec said her father kept horses when they lived there and I think he still had his trucking business.

At some point in her childhood, Cec was sent off to the United Church on Sunday mornings, often with an older brother or sister, sometimes by herself. From conversations I had with Cec, a long time ago near the beginning of our relationship, I was left with a vague impression of Cecile as a five- or six-year-old in a Sunday dress trotting down a residential sidewalk lined with towering oak trees to a red-brick cathedral.

I've only seen a few photos of Cec as a child. In each of them she is looking straight at the camera, a round solemn face, blonde hair in a bob. She was solid, self-contained. I could imagine her perched by herself on a hard pew paging through a hymnal laid open on the seat beside her. She liked the hymns and would have tried to sing along even though she struggled to carry a tune. If the sermon droned on, she'd slip out. No patience for boredom and she didn't like wearing a dress, preferred to be in hand-me-down play clothes, outside and out of sight.

Sometimes she'd slip into her dad's workshop and entertain herself while he worked. He didn't like it if she asked questions or touched his tools. But she was allowed to play with scraps of wood. If he was in a good mood he might pull a stool up to the counter, help her onto it, and hand her a small hammer, let her pound a nail. If his mood was dark she didn't stay. His rage could rise suddenly, especially if he'd been drinking. She became adept at keeping a calculated distance but wasn't always able to dodge him. More than once she went to school with bruises. She sat gingerly but without complaint. Complainers and whiners weren't tolerated.

Cec said she remembered her mother as towering and huge, broad in girth, a commanding presence. By the time I met Cec's mother she was stooped and bony. She smelled of cigarette smoke and an overpowering, flowery perfume. I had a hard time imagining her as physically imposing.

At fourteen, Cec moved in with Trevor, her oldest brother. They shared a small one-bedroom suite on the second floor of an older home owned by a stout, kerchiefed Polish woman. Cec's bed was the couch. During the day she went to school. School hadn't presented much of a challenge. She'd skipped two grades and graduated from high school at sixteen.

At night she worked in a factory assembling boxes. "I didn't need much sleep," she said.

She or Trev would make a big pot of soup or stew at the beginning of the week and as it dwindled, one of them would open a can of whatever was in the cupboard and dump that in.

"Fried lettuce is also pretty good."

"Fried lettuce?"

"Have you never tried it?"

"Why would you fry lettuce?"

"Because that's all there is. With a bit of butter, if you have it."

The Polish lady kicked them out after a couple of months. She didn't believe they were brother and sister. Thought they were living in sin.

I called Doreen on my way out to the farm to let her know I'd take care of chores in the morning, but yes, if she could do them tomorrow night, that would be great.

When we needed help with chores, we called Doreen. When it was time to send animals to auction, we called Doreen. When one of our chickens looked like it was sick, we called Doreen.

I was especially concerned about Ruby, one of our Dexter cows. Her belly was bulging with calf and she could deliver at any time. Doreen said she'd check in on her as often as she could. If Ruby needed help, Doreen would know what to do. Hank and Doreen had forty cows that they bred every year. During calving season in the spring, they checked their cows every couple of hours round the clock.

Our second spring on the farm, one of our Angus heifers, Violet, had her first calf while Cec and I were both at work. When we got home that night she was standing over the body of her baby, bellowing at him. He lay between her front hooves, eyes bulging, tongue hanging out, neck twisted. Violet had stood up when he was partway out and then sat back down again. Broke his neck.

A few weeks later Petunia had started to calve. It was early morning and Cec had gone out to do chores. I was just out of the shower and still dripping when I heard Cec call, "Petunia's having her baby! I might need your help."

I hurried to put on chore clothes and wondered, for a split second, whether I'd end up smelling like barnyard. I didn't want to have to take another shower.

The air was wet-cool, an early mid-April morning, clouds churning. Cec was in the large corral. She'd shooed out all the other cows and closed the gate. Petunia, the largest of our black Angus heifers, was lying on her side, heaving, nostrils flared. From the birth canal opening just below the pucker of her rectum protruded two small hooves.

"You're doing great, my girl." Cec held her voice to a whisper. "Shhh…" Cec put her finger to her lips as I opened the gate.

Petunia shifted her weight so that she was more upright. She grunted. Her sides heaved. Two knobby knees emerged. Then a small black nose.

"Atta girl!" Cec was smiling. We could see the outline of a calf head under the grey film of birth sack.

With Petunia's next huff, the calf's shoulders appeared.

"You ever seen this before?"

"No. You?"

Cec shook her head. Just then the shoulders slid out. The birth sack had torn open around the calf's face but it didn't look as though it was breathing. Petunia shifted her weight and planted her front hooves.

"She better not get up." Cec moved closer. Petunia pushed her front end up.

"Lie down girl." Cec's voice was low but firm. Petunia was trying to get up.

"C'mon!" Cec knelt down beside the half-birthed calf and grabbed hold of his hooves. "We have to hold her down!"

I dropped to my knees in the muck and wrapped my arms around the calf's skinny shoulders. Petunia grunted and heaved, trying to lift her back end up. We held on as tight as we could. The birth sack was slippery. I wrapped my arms around his torso and grabbed my hands together to hang on. Petunia's next heave pulled me flat onto the ground. Cec had ahold of the calf's front legs and was jerked face first into straw and muck.

"Don't let go!"

Petunia was on the move. If not for the weight of two grown humans creating a drag at her rear, she would already have been on her feet.

"Grab round the middle," I said to Cec. More of the calf's midsection emerged. My arms kept slipping. With locomotive power, Petunia generated a huffing, nostril-flared, forward motion that pulled us with her through the muck and slime.

"My god, she's strong." I tried to get a better grip for her next heave.

"Hang on!"

The next time Petunia heaved, the calf's hips popped free. His back legs slid out. Petunia grunted as she felt her rump swing sideways. She looked back, gave one more upwards heave and got to her feet.

The calf's eyes were open. As I unwrapped my arms from around his middle I saw his nostrils flare.

"Is he breathing?"

"His eyes are open."

Petunia took two unsteady steps toward her baby and sank down to the ground beside him. He was shivering. As Cec and I backed away. Petunia mooed at her baby and nudged him with her nose.

"That's the most beautiful sound I've ever heard," Cec whispered.

Petunia's big, rough tongue took random swipes at her calf's wet hide as she murmured at him in a single baritone note.

"I have to get to work."

"Yeah, well, actually, you need to be hosed down." Cec was grinning.

My face, hair, and all down my front were covered in muck. Somehow Cec had managed to keep her face and hair relatively untouched but we both looked like we'd been mud wrestling.

"You go get cleaned up. I'll stay, make sure he starts nursing." Cec turned back toward mama and baby. Petunia was still talking to her boy. "I could hang out here and listen to her all day."

Sometimes I open the doors to the small closet in our bedroom and bury my face in Cec's clothes—her Nygaard, Calvin Klein, Ralph Lauren. I close my eyes and for a few seconds I catch a fleeting glimpse of her face. Then she fades again and I can't conjure her—the angle of her jaw, the slope of her nose—no matter how tightly I squeeze my eyes.

I have resisted packing up her clothes. But it's been a year and my rational mind is insisting that a year is long enough. So I head out to the "little barn," a miniature hip roof barn that we had planned to turn into a cottage for summer guests. It's a plywood shell with a makeshift door that Cec built out of scrap wood. She painted the exterior red. I am using it as a storage shed. Thirteen containers filled with Cec's clothes are waiting there for me.

I open the containers and lift each item up for final inspection—her burgundy leather jacket, her plaid work shirts, her Ralph Lauren turtlenecks, her hot-pink dress. They are all too small for me. A few items I will keep—just because. Most I will donate.

I try on some of her shirts. A few of her pullovers fit. Cec used to buy shirts that were big on her. She liked rolling up her sleeves.

Some of these clothes I've never seen before—a sundress in bright neon colors, a pair of navy blue leather pants. From another life, I think, when she would squeeze herself into leather pants.

I hesitate when I come to Cec's chore coveralls. She had two pair. I hold up the light brown ones. They are worn, stained, ripped. The other pair is newer—a deep chocolate brown.

Cec wore her coveralls constantly. She'd change as soon as she got home from work. I saw her in those torn old coveralls more than I ever saw her in business suits or golf capris. Do I keep them? They don't fit me. The farm will be going up for sale.

This is one of those times I need to be tough, I tell myself. I put them both in the discard pile. I have an uneasy feeling that I will come to regret this decision.

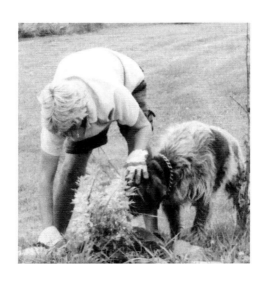

"It matters who you love"

Monday, February 28

I couldn't sleep. The emptiness of the farmhouse reverberated. The bed felt cold. I was up well before the sun, filled water dishes to the rim, gave extra oats to the horses who nipped and charged, trying to chase each other away from the trough.

They know about Cec, I thought. "Horses know stuff," Cec would say. She had an understanding with the horses and llamas, an unspoken communication. The smaller animals were less interesting as far as she was concerned, so they were mine. Not that we'd ever talked about it but I knew that's how it was. If you'd asked Cec she would have said the same, in different words, something like: "Lyn's too jumpy around the horses. She needs to relax."

We'd started with a small herd of Angus but slowly shifted over to Dexter cows and a Dexter bull. Dexters are a small breed and their calves are smaller, easier to deliver.

One day Doreen called Cec: did we want a Jersey calf? She thought we might like a good milk cow. Cec said we'd be right over.

Doreen coaxed Annie toward us by offering her a "sucky pail," a pail of milk with a nipple near the bottom. Annie sucked lustily. She was a lovely caramel brown with large brown eyes and tiny horn buds on her square forehead. She walked with the gangly walk of a Jersey, her ribs pronounced, hipbones jutting against sagging skin. While she sucked, she let us pat her. When she was finished, she tossed her head and pranced. We looked at each other and grinned. Annie was coming home with us.

I packed enough clothes for a week, threw in a deck of cards, a flashlight, a notebook and several books—one on herbal remedies that I thought Cec might want.

I called work and left a message for Euphemia who tracked vacation and sick days. I said that my husband had been taken to Emergency and I wouldn't be coming in.

My husband.

Because I wore the ring Cec had given me on the fourth finger of my left hand, Euphemia assumed I was married. I didn't want to lie but Cec was insistent.

"The minute I quit my job, I won't care," she said. "But the business world in Calgary is small. Someone will figure it out. I'm the only woman at my level in management and I have enough to deal with, without adding *that*."

"But it comes up. They ask."

"You don't have to answer. It's none of their business."

Easy for her to say. She was mistress of the side step, the master of evasion. She could redirect a conversation with a wrinkle of her nose and a blink of her eyes.

I, on the other hand, was a horrible liar, a fumbling evader. Cec said she was afraid to send me out into the world because I wore my feelings so plainly on my face, anyone could read me like an open book.

Which was my point exactly. *How did she think they wouldn't know?*

I hadn't tried to fool Tom. A week after I moved in with Cec I'd closed his office door and said, "I need to tell you something."

He'd leaned back in his chair. "Okay."

At 6' 3", Tom was the size and shape of a linebacker. He appreciated my facility with words, my ability to close sales, and liked it that I would disagree with him.

"I'm seeing someone."

"You don't have to—"

"Actually, I'm living with her."

"With *her*?"

I nodded.

He smiled, a slow, broad grin. "I think that's great!" When he smiled like that I could see the little boy in him, in the crinkles in the corners of his eyes. "If you're happy, then I'm happy for you."

"You can't tell anyone, not a word."

"I won't. And you didn't have to—"

"It's just in case."

"In case of what?"

"I don't know. It's just…hard not to say anything, to anyone, ever."

"Don't worry, I won't breathe a word."

I believed him.

Cec said I was being naive. "You never tell them anything they can use against you. Especially someone you work with. And especially your boss! You might have a great relationship now, but you never know."

I walked as fast as I could, without actually running, down the hospital hallway. As I rounded the last corner I could see that there were people in Cec's room. A large frame blocked my view—almost as tall as me, with broad shoulders wearing baggy cords, a dark blue turtleneck, and a knitted vest.

The broad shoulders turned to me. Her face was square-ish with straight dark hair cut in the shape of a football helmet. A hospital ID badge hung around her neck.

Dr. Somers, from the Emergency Ward the night before, was at Cec's bedside. She was with another doctor. They stepped past the large woman with the ID badge and Somers nodded at me. When they were gone, I held out my hand. "Hi, I'm Lyn."

Her grip was firm. "I'm Marion. The chaplain."

I didn't know whether the doctors had interrupted Marion's conversation with Cec? What I knew with certainty was that the moment Marion's squarish frame had appeared in the doorway, Cec had decided she didn't like her. I'd seen Cec respond this way to women before, especially if they had short, cropped hair and a stocky or athletic, build.

Cec had said once, early in our relationship, that she didn't think of herself as lesbian.

"How can you be with me and not be lesbian?" I'd asked, a little surprised. I had no doubt that she was attracted to me. Maybe she thought that a lesbian was only ever attracted to women? Or had never been with a man?

"That's just how it is," was all she would say.

Marion's eyes were kind. "You are...her sister?"

"I'm her partner."

"Oh. Uh. Hi. When Cecile filled out the admission form she checked the box for spiritual care?" Marion stepped into the room.

"Now's not a really good time," Cec said. "They're going to send me for more tests."

"Okay. Well. I'll come back later then."

Marion left and Cec said, "I wanted someone from spiritual care but..."

"Not her?"

"Can't they send someone else?"

"Why don't you want her?"

"Why do you think?"

"She might *not* be a dyke."

Cec lowered her head, raised her eyebrows, gave me an

"oh puh-lease" look over the rim of her glasses. There would be no point in trying to convince her otherwise.

"What did the doctors have to say?"

"I've been assigned a resident that works in this ward. She'll come by later."

"Did they say anything about test results?"

"No, just that they're sending me for more."

"But they must have an idea—"

"I think they know—"

"Know what?"

"Did you call Doreen about chores?"

Cec was purposely changing the subject. I hated the sense I had that she knew more than she was letting on.

"I called Doreen this morning before I came in. And I moved bales."

"Are you going into work?"

"I called in."

"What did you say?"

"That my husband was taken into Emergency last night."

"Your husband?"

"My husband."

Cec smiled. "Good girl." She motioned me closer. "I need your help." She pushed back her blankets. "Get me out of this bed," she said. "If I'm going to get better, I have to keep moving."

I hesitated. I wasn't so sure.

"Are you going to help me?"

I took hold of her elbow as she wriggled her legs over the side of the bed.

"Wait, I have to unplug your IV machine." I pulled the plug out of the socket and wrapped the cord around the monitor. "You can hold onto the pole."

She grabbed the pole with one hand and took my arm with the other. I matched my steps to hers as we moved slowly toward the door. I wasn't sure where she thought we were headed.

We were looking at cottages on one- and two-acre lots.

We had just bought a house in Calgary, a new car for me, an SUV for her, a sofa and love seat, a new bed, a band saw and a mitre saw to add to Cec's collection of woodworking tools. We were on a spree, the domestic ritual of acquisition, each new item adding substance. Our purchases felt like gifts to each other, but not exactly, more like bricks in the foundation of a life we were building together. And now Cec had the idea that we should buy a property, a weekend getaway.

The cottages were small and separated from each other by a row of spindly evergreens. The water was never a real incentive, covered in algae or ringed with bulrush, the beach a fifteen-minute walk away or barely visible through dense brush, accessible along a path that Cec was certain would require a machete to clear.

The further we drove west, into the foothills and the shadow of the Rocky Mountains, the deeper the furrow in her brow.

"Too much snow," she said.

"Snow?"

"They get a lot more snow here. The warm wind comes over the mountains and dumps all its moisture here. And there are more wild animals."

I wasn't sure why we had come this far west. My preference was prairie to forest, but I'd already said that to her. Mountains made me claustrophobic.

"Bears. Cougars. Predators," she said. "They eat small dogs."

The small cottages were too small. The big ones too palatial. "Like owning a second house," Cec said. "All we need is a place where you can write and I can chop wood, take the dogs for long walks. We don't need a lake. A river would be nice."

I made a mental note to get Cec a machete for her birthday, a real one, for clearing underbrush. Whether or not she ever used it, she'd like the idea of having one. She had already said that she wanted a chainsaw, to fell dead trees. She had never used a chainsaw but that wouldn't deter her. She would climb any tree, cut into any branch at any height. Her fearlessness terrified me.

We'd been driving country roads and checking the local listings for nine months, off and on. Nothing was jumping out at us. Or, rather, nothing was jumping out at Cec. We'd drive by a place and she'd shake her head. I'd nod in agreement. To be honest, none of the cottages or lakes or patches of underbrush waiting to be cleared had whispered my name either.

"I'd like a workshop," Cec said. "Doesn't have to be very large but heated so I can work out there year-round."

We were in Linden, a predominantly Mennonite hamlet about an hour northeast of Calgary. Cec had bought the *Capital*, the local paper, at Esau's Gas and was reading through the listings on the back page as she sipped tea. I was eating homemade Mennonite food, perogies and farmer sausage, at the Country Cousins.

Linden was almost too far from Calgary for a daily commute but the land was beautiful, gently rolling. Every few miles we passed another Holdemon church. The Holdemons are an ultra-conservative Mennonite sect. The women wear flower print dresses and put their hair into little black "bun holders." My grandparents weren't Holdemon, but my grand-mother had always worn a flower print dress and one of those black bun holders. I had relatives that were Holdemon and I was grateful that I'd been born on the more liberal side of the Mennonite divide.

"This one," Cec said, tapping her finger on a photo of a small white farmhouse. It looked as though it had started out as a small rectangular two storey and then had an addition built out to one side. There was a deck off the front. It looked very plain. I read the ad while Cec called the realtor.

"Forty acres?" I had just swallowed a mouthful of perogies with a peppery cottage cheese filling. "We don't need forty acres."

She shrugged, "There's a creek that runs through the pasture and there's a barn. Could be my workshop. We're out here anyway. Might as well have a look."

It was October, a Saturday of bright sunlight that warmed orange leaves to a yellow glow. The realtor called back. She couldn't show the place that day but we could drive by and have a look at the property, just as long as we didn't drive into the yard. The owners were adamant about showings by appointment only.

Six miles south on the 806, then west on the 587 for another five or six miles, through Sunnyslope and then north on the next Range Road. Cec was writing down directions. Did she know where Sunnyslope was? No.

Sunnyslope turned out to be a small collection of houses and trailers at the bottom of a gully. A train had once stopped on a daily basis in Sunnyslope to transport workers to their jobs in the larger centres. All that was left of the railroad was an old rail bed and piles of ties, the tracks long since removed.

Just past the Sunnyslope Community Centre—a mustard-yellow building with a brown tin roof and no windows—we turned right onto a road with a sign that said, "No Exit." Half a mile up the dead end road and off to the right sat the white farmhouse we'd seen in the ad.

We stopped when we came to the driveway, about a quarter of a mile long. A green metal gate guarded the entrance. It was closed, and padlocked.

"They're serious about no visitors." Cec unfolded her map. "Here's the Kneehill, the creek that runs through Sunnyslope. Some of those forty acres must be down in the gully." Cec turned the vehicle around. "Let's go see what the back side of this property looks like."

We drove back through Sunnyslope and turned north on a gravel road that ran along the bottom of the gully. We crossed a cattle grate and found ourselves driving through a herd of black heifers, some on the right, and others to the left, of the road. They continued to graze, unconcerned. We could see the white farmhouse and the barn at the top of the ridge, and the way the land sloped down to the creek. Once we had passed the cows, Cec stopped the car. We got out and made our way across a stretch of pasture, then up an embankment and across an old rail bed that ran parallel to the road.

We came to a barbed-wire fence. "This must be the end of the property," I said. We didn't have a map or anything to indicate the boundary of the forty acres, but it made sense. The fence enclosed a rectangular piece of prairie that stretched all the way up to the buildings perched on the upper ridge of the gully. Forty acres is a lot of land, and the farmyard seemed very far away.

The land rolled. We couldn't see the creek from where we stood. I lifted the barbed wire for Cec so she could crawl through. Sage grew everywhere, small bushes as well as the kind that looked more like an herb and grew in tufts and clusters. Gophers popped out of their holes to chatter at us. As we walked toward the farmyard the ridge loomed larger and larger and I could see that the land fell away more sharply than I'd thought.

As we got closer, we could see that the creek was wider

than it had looked from the road: thirty or maybe forty feet across, and banks six to ten feet high that sloped down to the water. It had carved a winding path through the bottom of the gully. In some sections the water was high and wide as a small river, but as we walked we could see that there were places where the creek was almost dry. At one of the low spots we saw tire tracks across the creek bed.

I couldn't see the house anymore but the barn sat very close to the edge of the ridge. I shielded my eyes from the sun as I looked up. We wouldn't walk up the ridge. That would put us right on the farmyard and we didn't have an appointment.

"Cec, look!" A row of black cows were standing along the top of the ridge looking down at us.

"Hi girls!" Cec called, and waved. The cows didn't move. "They must be the watch cows."

Some kind of prairie farm madness took hold of us both that day. I don't know when it happened for Cec. For me it happened while we stood there on the stubble of uneven prairie beside a wide-mouthed stagnating creek. As I stood, shielding my eyes from the sun and watching the cows watch us, I fell in love.

A young nurse with curly brown hair and matronly hips entered the room.

"This is Lorraine," Cec said.

The nurse nodded in my direction and said to Cec, "On a scale of one to ten?" The way she said it, I could tell they'd had this conversation before.

"About a four."

"You want to stay at five milligrams?"

"I want to go down."

"But five—"

"—makes me nauseous."

"I could give you Gravol."

Cec shook her head. "Gravol makes me sleepy."

"You could try Maxeran. I can add it to your IV."

"We can try."

"I think you should stay at five—"

"2.5."

Lorraine smiled. "Okay, 2.5. I'll be right back."

She left and Cec said, "She's good. I felt bad for my nurse last night."

"Were you a miserable patient?"

"Me? Of course not." Cec feigned surprise. She pointed toward her roommate on the other side of the curtain and whispered, "She kept calling. A couple times he didn't get there fast enough and—" Cec pinched her nose. "Ew!"

"You had a male nurse?"

"Lawrence." Her head fell back against the pillow. Her

eyes closed. "I don't like having a fuzzy head." A moment later. "I liked him."

"Who?"

"Lawrence. He has warm hands."

A male nurse. I hadn't considered that possibility. But of course I should have. That would suit her perfectly, especially if he was young.

Cec wasn't the kind of beauty that made men turn their heads or stop talking mid-sentence. She knew this. But she also understood how to draw their attention. Something in the way she held her head, moved her hips, narrowed her eyes.

I knew what it felt like to want to move closer. I was drawn to her confidence, to her quirky humour, her unwavering calm, her genuine curiousity.

I was pretty sure that the young men that worked for her often suffered a similar sense of magnetic attraction and mild bewilderment. What was she offering? What did she want?

Her latest protégé at the office (and she usually had at least one on the go) was Damien, her manager of ocean freight. He had a boyish charm and a knack for diversionary humour, especially when he'd screwed up.

Cec said he would enter her office without knocking, and plunk himself into a chair. She'd keep her head down, pen scribbling, pages flipping. She didn't shoo him out. His chatter was useful—project updates and bits of gossip.

"You could take a break you know," he'd say, leaning back in the chair.

She let him get away with a casual tone, a calculated move.

"Can I get you a tea?" He was consumed with his own enthusiasm, unconcerned with her lack of response.

She would look up, over the rim of her glasses. "Are you looking for something to do?"

He'd grin. He'd made her look up. Not that it really mattered. He assumed that his presence necessarily meant he had moved into the centre of her attention, eye contact or not.

"Did you watch Tiger at the Masters this weekend?"

Cec nodded.

"A twenty-two stroke lead!"

Cec knew she couldn't afford to let him to settle into golf banter. "Yes, he was good."

"Good? Just good?"

"Damien!" Time to dial him back. "There is something I need you to do." She could tell from the sag of his shoulders that her tone had had the desired effect. "I'm working on a quote for a shipment of pipe to Turkey. I just got the numbers from the steamship lines. I need you to write it up."

"I can do that!"

"Right away, please."

She'd double-check his work. He'd like having an excuse to come back into her office.

One Friday evening Cec said, out of nowhere, "Damien asked me to go with him to the company Christmas party."

I was washing dishes, my back to her. "He did?"

"He came into my office…" I thought about turning around so I could see her face, but I already knew from the tone of her voice that his question had pleased her, "…and asked whether I was going with anyone."

I turned to look at her. *Did my eyes give away my—what was it—jealousy? Was that what she was after?*

"Men make statements," she'd said, in a conversation about office politics, "and women ask questions, very sincere questions through which they telegraph their motivations and desires. They expect a sincere answer. Men will throw out a statement as though it's fact even when they know it's utter bullshit, just to see how others respond. They get the information they need without showing their own hand."

Was this a test?

I turned back to the dishes in the soapy water without saying anything.

"I think he was fishing to see whether I'm still with Anthony." She was beside me now, had picked up a tea towel.

Anthony. Tony. The tennis player. Cec had taken Tony with her to the Christmas party the year before.

"He offered to pick me up, since we were both going anyway." It was evident she was pleased by his interest, and his offer.

"And you said…?" I let my question hang as I glanced at her face. She had turned to open a cupboard to put a plate away and I couldn't see her eyes.

"I said that it wouldn't be appropriate."

The flush in my cheeks and the clench of my jaw was less about Damien asking her to the party and more about her not asking me, and knowing she never would.

"His question was harmless, Lyn. It didn't mean anything."

Which wasn't true. I kept my head down, my hands in the sudsy water, wondering why she had told me.

To demonstrate her desirability?

To prove she doesn't keep secrets.

Cec took off her tank top and sandwiched it between her bum and the seat of the garden tractor. She wasn't wearing a bra, but who would care? She squinted to keep dust and bugs from flying into her eyes. When she switched to the push mower for around the house, she tossed her tank top onto the deck. While she mowed, I weeded, on my hands and knees, the sun hot on my neck.

The pail beside me was heavy with weed greens for the chickens when Cec came up behind me.

"You don't have to get every single one!" I could tell by the tone of her voice that she was standing with her hands on her hips.

"If I don't I'll have to do this all over again in a few days."

What did it matter how I weeded the garden? I kept pulling weeds.

"It's like you become obsessed."

I wanted to say, *And you always have an opinion!* but I bit back the words.

Another time, when she'd been on my case about watering the flower beds with a spray wand (she thought the beds got a better soaking with the sprinkler) I'd said, "I'm fine with your critiques and criticisms as long as you also let me know when I've done a good job."

Her response was immediate: "I don't want to have to pat you on the back all the time."

All the time?

I just about said, *Once would be nice,* but there wasn't any point. I didn't say anything, didn't look at her, kept watering.

The chestnut brown of Cec's skin had deepened during the day. No hint of red on her anywhere. The back of my neck felt hot to the press of my hand.

The sun had wearied us both. After a dinner of salad and watermelon she poured two glasses of ice water and we sank into lawn chairs on the front deck.

"Every time I look at that tree, I think about how it needs to be pruned," Cec said, pointing to the oak in the front yard. "And the lilac bushes."

I was about to say, *But not now*, when she said, "Don't worry, not right this minute."

"It looks so great when it's just been cut," I said, holding up my glass in a toast to her efforts and felt the cold slide all the way down my throat into my stomach. I was about to lean my head back and close my eyes when she said, "So, when did you first know?"

"Know what?"

"That you were attracted to women."

I looked at her. Did she really want me to answer? She had been minimally forthcoming about her past relationships, and hadn't showed much interest in hearing about mine. But she looked so relaxed, leaning back in her chair, eyes almost falling shut.

"Anna," I said.

"Anna?"

"I met her when I was at the folk school. In Denmark."

"Was she a student?"

"She lived in the same town as my Danish host family."

"You were attracted to her."

From the moment I met Anna, I was instantly aware of her every movement, where she was in the room, whom she was talking with.

"I had no idea then that it was possible for me to fall in love with a woman."

"But you did."

"Only in retrospect. I didn't realize at the time."

Cec leaned back in her chair, probably thinking about Anna, like I was. After a bit she said, "You have this little world inside your head that you keep all to yourself."

I wanted to say, *And you don't?* but instead I said, "That was a long time ago."

"You're still attracted to her."

I took a deep breath. There wasn't anything I could say that wouldn't get me in trouble. Cec was sure that I was attracted to everyone and anyone. We'd be watching TV—I use the word "watching" loosely, Cec rarely ever sat down to watch TV but she often put it on as background noise—and she'd look up from her computer over the rim of her glasses and say, "You like him," pointing to the lead guy on the TV show *JAG*. I would deny, up and down, but it didn't matter. She started calling him my "boyfriend," in a tone that was only half-teasing.

If I admitted an attraction to Anna, it would be a problem. If I denied my attraction, Cec wouldn't believe me anyway.

"Have I shown you her picture?" I knew I hadn't shown Cec my photos of Anna, or the notes she had written me in her pointy scrawl.

"She was beautiful," Cec said, not because she knew but to see how I would react.

"And elusive. She wouldn't talk to me at all. For months."

"You liked that."

Although I didn't want to admit it, Cec was right. Anna gave off an air of aloofness but her eyes were often sad.

"You're still in love with her."

"That was a long time ago."

"Doesn't matter how long—"

"She got married."

Cec didn't say anything.

"I haven't seen her or talked to her for years."

Cec scanned the horizon. "I didn't realize—"

"You asked me when I knew. That's when I knew."

"Obviously I should have asked sooner." She stood up. "She's a part of my past, Babe. We all have history."

"Yes, but I didn't realize that you were still in love."

"I'm not!"

"Don't lie to me!"

"She lives on another continent."

"Doesn't matter."

"It doesn't matter what I say."

"It matters who you love." She turned and walked into the house. A moment later I heard the back door open, then slam.

Cec's new doctor swayed as she walked. "Margaret Kendrick," she said, with a smile.

"Cecile." Cec tried to sit up straighter.

This new doctor was a mother of teenagers, I thought. She probably still made their lunches.

Dr. Kendrick flipped through the pages on her clipboard. "You're scheduled for surgery on Wednesday, March 2." She seemed to be speaking to herself more than to Cec. "Your surgery is scheduled for here. That keeps everything simple." She flipped the papers back. "We're hoping the surgery will provide some answers. All I can tell you is that we don't know anything for sure."

Still nothing? It never took this long on television.

"How is your pain, on a scale of one to ten?"

"A three, sometimes five. Morphine makes me…blurry… not in my buddy."

Kendrick didn't seem surprised by Cec's incoherence.

"We're also giving you Maxeran, which should help with the nausea."

"I don't lick dopey…having feeler…dreams."

"You're having bad dreams?"

Cec nodded.

"And you don't like them."

Cec shook her head.

"We could bring you down to 2.5 mils and see how that works."

"Morph een dow en." Her voice was thin, high-pitched.

"I'll put a note in your chart that you can indicate your

own level, up to ten milligrams."

"No ten!" Cec shook her head vigorously. Her cheeks were flushed.

"Just in case." Kendrick scribbled. "And how are your bowel movements?"

I waited for her to respond. Nothing.

"Her bowels have never been great," I said.

"Eh!" Cec waggled a finger at me.

"That true?" Kendrick asked Cec.

Cec's head fell back. She was struggling to keep her eyes open.

"It's true," I said. "Even if she doesn't want to admit it."

"Morphine slows all physical functions, including the bowels. I'll put you on a stool softener."

"Seno…" Cec said, and then her eyes rolled up into the back of her head. All I could see were the white undersides of her eyeballs.

"Senokot?" Kendrick asked, watching.

"Her mom was on it."

Cec's eyes rolled forward. She took a deep breath. "Senokot."

"I'll order Senokot for you, and also a laxative." Kendrick kept writing. "A mild one."

Kendrick left and an orderly arrived to take Cec down for another X-ray. I remained sitting after she was gone. I knew I should go in to work. But what would I do there? I couldn't focus. I hoped Euphemia had let Tom know. I thought he would have called me by now. Maybe just as well.

Cec had called her office, told them she was in the hospital and would have to have minor surgery. They shouldn't expect her for a couple of days. Then she'd called Franz, the sales VP, at the head office in Toronto. She'd told him the same. Called it "a minor setback," said she expected to be out again in a few days. And she didn't want anyone to send flowers. No visitors. She asked Franz to please let everyone know. She didn't want any of them to see her in her flimsy hospital nightie. I expect that she also didn't want any of them to meet me.

I left her room and walked past the nurses' station then down the ward hallway lined with wheelchairs and pink vinyl recliners. I'd seen nurses rolling the recliners into the rooms for patients to use as an alternative to lying in bed. I often saw visitors sitting in these wheelchairs waiting for a nurse to finish, or taking a break but wanting to stay close. *Why so many?* The entire hallway lined with them. At the end of the hall there was another room filled with more wheelchairs. These were the broken ones, missing footrests, seats and wheels. I stopped for a moment. They looked forlorn, like I felt, with nowhere to go.

As I turned to continue my walk around the loop of the ward, I had a sudden sensation of Cec coming toward me pushing a wheelbarrow piled high with compost. I stopped in the middle of the hallway. I could see her grinning, her eyes squinting in a dare. She would come straight at me. I'd plant my feet. Who would move first? I would. She never gave way. But if I timed it right, I could grab her around her middle. She'd let go of the wheelbarrow handles as I lifted her and swung her around. The wheelbarrow would drop, rocking from side to side as it settled.

The hallway seemed to be moving, a slow revolution. I steadied myself against the wall with my fingertips and kept walking.

I was six when my father applied for and was awarded a teaching position in Norway House, an Aboriginal reservation in northern Manitoba, a small town located on the northernmost tip of Lake Winnipeg, inaccessible by road except over frozen ice in the winter. When we arrived, in the fall of 1972, Norway House was the reserve with the highest rate of alcohol consumption per capita in Canada. My guess is that hairspray and Lysol consumption were also at an all-time high. The daily diets of the kids I went to school with included fewer fresh fruit and veggies, and contained less meat than any other school-age group of children in Canada. From what I observed, most of them survived on what they could steal from the Hudson's Bay store: chips, pop, Kool-Aid crystals. They lived in houses built by the government, window openings covered with plastic, little or no furniture, no indoor plumbing. I'd catch glimpses—as a front door would open and close—of wood floors and bare walls.

I was the only white kid in grades one to three, and since these three grades had recess together I was effectively the sole white face on the playground, and also tall for my age. I made a perfect target.

The boys would swarm me, moving as a pack. One of the big boys would take me down from behind. The others would close in.

I learned quickly how to roll into a ball, wrap my arms around my head, and (of greatest importance) make no sound. No tears.

The rapid-fire kicks would lessen, the punches subside. They'd back off, or a teacher would pull them off.

I'd get up and brush the dirt off my clothes, refuse to make eye contact.

My brother fared better. He was a year and a half younger, in kindergarten, the same class as Shane, the Hudson's Bay manager's son.

"Just kick 'em in the face," Shane said to James. The Aborginal kids thought it was a novelty to watch a white kid sit on a toilet. They'd look under the door, pointing and giggling, or climb up and peer over top.

"Just kick 'em in the face!" Shane was matter-of-fact and so was James when he reported to Mom after school.

"But you don't actually kick them!" My mother was horrified.

"Yup, I do," James said, his mouth full of chocolate chip cookie. "I do what Shane says."

James's greatest injury was to the tips of his fingers. His kindergarten comrades, Shane included, would collect the used cigarette butts on the playground at recess and try to light them. James burned his fingers accepting the wrong end of a lit butt.

He also expanded his vocabulary.

"Fuckshitpastor!"

"What did you say?" My father looked up from his dinner.

James obliged. "Fuck. Shit. Pastor."

"Pastor?" Dad was trying not to laugh. "I think he means bastard."

"Yup." James nodded. "Pastor!"

Mom was shaping the dough into loaves and plopping them into bread pans. "One thing we did right was taking you out of school."

Yes, they had finally taken me out of school.

We lived in a row of townhouses built especially for

teachers at the edge of the schoolyard. Every recess I ran home and begged my mother to let me stay home.

No. She was firm. I couldn't miss school.

"That was a time when you didn't consider taking your child out of school. It just wasn't done. No one was home-schooling."

But your six-year-old child runs home at every recess, at every possible opportunity, and pleads with you to let her stay home, and you wipe away her tears and keep sending her back?

My dad taught in a classroom on the second floor. The window of his classroom overlooked the playground. He saw me down there sometimes, he said. Was I standing up, I wondered, or smashed down in the dirt? I didn't ask. If he saw me, why didn't he come get me? Somehow I knew it wasn't possible. Even if he wanted to, for some reason he couldn't.

As unfortunate circumstance would have it, my grade two teacher was Mrs. Korzonowski, a stout, plump matron who, mysteriously, came to school each day with a different hair colour.

Wigs. It took me a while, but I figured it out.

Mrs. Korzonowski lacked the skills necessary to manage twenty-nine running, yelling seven-, eight-, nine- and ten-year-olds (a number of my classmates were repeating grade two for the second or third time). I sat at a desk at the back of the class with my head bowed over my reader or my math book. Adding up numbers brought a small measure of comfort. Tiny columns of logic. A method for arriving at a solution. An answer that made some sense.

I refused to look up. Not when I was bumped, or pinched, or my pencil pulled out of my hand. I shut out the squeals, and the rising pitch of Mrs. Korzonowski's agitation. Eventually she would pull out her strap and march up and down the rows of desks, flicking. Her ability to hit her target had earned her a certain measure of respect. The pandemonium would subside.

"What are you doing?" A hand would jiggle my pencil. Another hand would push my eraser onto the floor. Small fingers would pull at the fine hairs on my arm, curiosity more than malice, often two or three of them at a time, sometimes stroking my arm, sometimes a pinch. I didn't look up, and I didn't flinch.

Eventually I stopped running home at recess. Apparently I also stopped talking. Mom said I'd sit at the breakfast table and eat a few mouthfuls of porridge, my eyes brimming with tears. Some would spill over. I'd wipe them away before I left for school.

One day my mother saw me walking home from school across the bare field between our house and the schoolyard. I was glancing behind me every few steps. In the distance a group of three or four kids, a couple years older than me, were heading in my direction. Mom said I moved like a soldier on a battlefield, the way I dove behind a pile of stones and lay there on my belly. The kids stopped. They headed off toward the Hudson's Bay store. I got up, dusted myself off, and ran the rest of the way home.

Was that when my parents took me out of school?

No, I think it was after Christmas.

I didn't want to go to the Christmas concert. My grade two class was supposed to sing a song. I didn't want to wear a dress or sing about goodwill. My parents insisted. I put on the red dress that my mother had made especially for the occasion.

All the classes gathered in the lunch area while we waited for our turn on stage. Someone set up the projector and got a big spool of film spinning. A Western. Sweaty white men on horses carrying guns, their shirts unbuttoned. I remember being surprised by how much hair they had on their chests.

One of the men hit the other one. Then he pulled a

brand out of a hot fire and pressed it into the guy's hairy chest. Skin bubbled up. The man screamed. I covered my eyes and rocked back and forth, trying to block out his screams.

I felt a hand on my shoulder. Dad. He'd come to check on me. He pulled me to my feet, picked me up, and carried me out of there even though I was too big to be carried.

"If you're just going to sit there and stare at me," Cec said, "I don't want you here!"

Don't want me here?

"I want to be around people that are normal."

"Normal? What about this is normal?"

"You're hovering and you're jumpy and you look at me like I'm *special*." She said *special* with the Danish pronunciation. In Danish *special* means not quite right in the head.

"I thought you were…" There wasn't any point. She could lie there with her *normal* roommate and breathe in the *normal* stink of someone else's shit. If she wanted me to leave, I could leave. And never come back. Ever. Is that what she wanted?

I left the room and walked the loop of the ward—long strides to shake off my agitation—down one hallway past the shower room and cleaning room and back up the other side.

Am I nuts? I was muttering under my breath, furious with her, and with myself. *She tells me to leave and I stay close.* Moth to the proverbial flame: get close, get burned, fly away, return, repeat.

I walked the loop a second time, slowing, until I stopped in front of one of the many wheelchairs lining the hallway, pushed open the armrests, and sat down.

I'd told her once that she was abusive. I braced myself for her fury but instead she sounded defeated. "How could you say that? Everything I do, all of it, is for you, for us."

In that moment, disarmed by what seemed like her

genuine surprise and hurt at my unfair accusation, I believed her and felt bad.

Later I realized she hadn't apologized. Her response had been a justification, a sadness-infused outrage.

"You want to know what I think?" she'd said in another one of those standoffs where I wasn't backing down. We were out near the barn.

I didn't actually care what she thought.

"I think you're gearing up to leave and you want to dump it all on me."

"No!" My response was instant, a reflex. "No." The second time more deliberate. "I don't want to dump it all on you." Something inside me meant it. "And no, I don't want to leave." I felt the words form in my mouth but it was as though someone else was saying them.

Cec had said once, "If we ever split, we won't do it cruel, right?"

I nodded. We wouldn't do it cruel, but it would be massively uncomfortable. She would refuse to speak to me or look at me. Her silence would harden. I would have to force myself to walk into another room to stop myself from trying to negotiate a return. There would be no point in talking.

"What are you doing?" Cec's eyes opened, her head raised.

"Filling out this form, for a phone and TV." I bent down to get my wallet from my purse.

Cec said, "Give them my credit card."

"Yours?"

She nodded, "If something happens, you won't have to pay."

If something happens.

We weren't married, couldn't legally get married. We didn't have any joint accounts. My name wasn't on any of her credit cards. I wasn't certain but I thought there was a strong possibility I couldn't be held liable for her debts.

I pulled her credit card out of my wallet, wrote her number in the blank space and handed her the clipboard. She waved me away.

"You sign," she said.

"Me? It's your card."

"Sign my name."

"But you—"

"They won't know the difference."

"Yes they will."

The first time I met Anna, she walked up to me after a church service, extended her hand and said, with a smile, "*God dag, og velkommen.*" I managed, "*God dag.*" She was slender, on the tall side of average, with a tightly wound energy that spilled into continuous movement. As she offered me her hand, she leaned back and studied me with her wide-set blue eyes. She smiled but seemed uncertain what to do next as she shook my hand. Her grip was firm. There was strength in the way she held herself and a sensuous fragility in her long, cool fingers and finely chiseled, high-set cheekbones. She repeated her greeting. "Welcome…to…Herning," in slow, deliberate English, then turned away. She gave me the distinct impression that she had no intention of ever speaking to me again.

I was eighteen years old and had come to Mariager, a small town in Denmark to attend the Pinsevækkelsens Højskole for a year. The Højskole was a folk school run by the Danish Pentecostal Church.

For months, Anna would smile and nod as I passed. If we found ourselves in the same small cluster in the foyer after a service, she would speak Danish so rapidly she knew I wouldn't be able to follow.

I kept her in my sights, stayed as close as I could. I'd sit in a pew where I could watch her fingers play across the piano keys, her shoulder leaning into the music. Her twin sister, Lisette, who resembled Anna only mildly, was more willing to speak English and would offer up polite conversation while Anna stood by in silence or slipped away.

The Jensen twins were the youngest of eleven kids and their father, a short, round and overly jovial man, handed out the programs each Sunday at the doors to the sanctuary. There was no slipping past him and he seemed to like the idea of greeting the Canadian with extra gusto.

I'd just extricated myself from a particularly vociferous greeting when I heard Anna's voice in my ear, "*Min far kan lide dig.*" I'd been in Denmark for several months and understood enough Danish to know what she'd said: "My father likes you." By the time I turned, she was gone.

Then one evening after a youth service, I sensed someone beside me and turned to find Anna.

"I have English exam at school tomorrow," she said, looking straight ahead as though she wasn't actually talking to me.

I was surprised, and pleased.

"I could help you," I said, trying to sound nonchalant. "We could practice."

"Thank you. But I am, how you say...*på Dansk det hedder 'flaug.'*"

"Embarrassed?"

She nodded, "I am embarrassed. Since my English, it is bad."

"Your English isn't—"

"You talk in Dansk with no accent. I not know how it is...*muligt?*"

"Possible."

"How it is possible you have not accent." There was a lift of admiration in her voice. Then her voice dropped again, "It makes me know how I am—"

"But you're—"

She turned her face away.

"Is there something? Are you okay?" I'd sensed this sadness in her before, when she'd sit at the piano, hands in her lap, listening to Søren, the pastor, give his opening greetings, waiting for her cue.

"Carston," she whispered, leaning in close. I almost didn't hear, and wouldn't have known what she'd said if I didn't already know.

Carston, the son of Søren and Leila. Leila who could never hold her tongue and said whatever came to her mind without a shred of sensitivity for situation. Carston had dark curly hair and smiling blue eyes. He was the conductor of the youth choir and, like Anna, gave off an air of untouchability. I had heard that Anna liked Carston (in quiet titters, because teenage girls can't help themselves) and I had heard that Søren didn't like Anna, no explanation given, except maybe that it had something to do with Anna's rotund, obnoxious father.

"It's hard for me," she said, "because we spend so much time together, at the choir practices and in the youth group. At first that is good and I am liking him and we have it nice."

A tremble of emotion rippled through her, and she struggled to pull it back. Without looking up, she said, "But something happens. Maybe someone says to him something. I don't know. He stops looking to me. I think everyone can see. And I must smile, in the front, by the piano."

I took a small step closer and bent my head toward hers, to shield her from the sightlines of all the perpetually curious.

"Someone always watches," she said, with a shake of her head. Then her composure returned. She attempted a smile. "Sometimes in school my... how you say... 'kommerater'?"

"Your friends?"

"My friends, they say they can see how I am. I can't hide from my face."

The rituals of the Pentacostal Church in Denmark were familiar. I'd grown up in the conservative predictability of a Mennonite Brethren congregation. The Pentecostals in

Denmark weren't so different really, except for the Gifts of the Spirit: the speaking in tongues, laying on of hands, words of prophecy. Time was allotted in the service for the expression of the Gifts. Spontaneous outbursts were not encouraged.

Mennonites believe that the Gifts of the Spirit were for biblical times but not for the present day. During my last years of high school my mother had begun to question this. Why would God's Spirit change? Why would He withdraw His Gifts? She attended charismatic revival services, lifted her hands in the air during worship, swayed back and forth. Sometimes I went with her. I liked the upbeat music, found myself speaking in tongues—the babble of baby syllables. Not so mysterious really. Once I even fell over in the Spirit, straight back, my body stiff as a tree trunk. I don't remember hitting the floor.

A visiting evangelist suggested that I might want to consider attending a Pentecostal folk school he'd heard about. In Denmark. It was like a bible school, he said, but no tests or exams, more of a cultural experience.

"When you come in the weekend, you come to me," Anna said.

I began staying with Anna whenever I went to Herning.

One Friday night I arrived at her parents' house while she was still out. She'd said that if I got there before her I should just go in, the door would be unlocked.

I went upstairs to her bedroom, changed into my pajamas, brushed my teeth, crawled into bed. I was tired but determined to stay awake.

I didn't hear the door or Anna's steps up the stairs. When I opened my eyes she was in the room, breathless and rosy-cheeked. I raised myself onto an elbow as she said, "*Hej min egen!*" Before I could answer, she bent down and kissed me. On the lips. She smiled, took off her jacket. She was bubbly, brimming. Something had happened—a look or a smile from one of the many hopefuls vying for her attention. I lay back listening to her chatter, basking in her effervescence, the stir of her kiss.

She pulled off her clothing until she was naked except for her pale purple cotton panties, clinging to the points of her hipbones, loose around the concave of her tummy. From where I lay I had an unobstructed view of her tanned legs, evenly rounded breasts, nipples red-brown. She smiled down at me as she brushed her hair into a ponytail and pulled a T-shirt over her head. She climbed into bed beside me. "It was a lovely evening," she said, turning to me, "and better even, now you are here."

Her eyes closed. Her breathing slowed. She rolled onto her side, her back to me. I closed my eyes and imagined my body curled around hers.

When I woke in the middle of the night Anna's hand was resting on my arm. She was curled in a ball beside me, her head almost touching my shoulder. I lay perfectly still, inhaling the rosemary-orange scent of her hair.

I was sitting at my mother's kitchen table watching her chop cabbage. Her hands were red from scrubbing carrots, fingertips purple from chopping beets. She cut the cabbage in half and laid the flat side on the counter, cut it lengthwise again and chopped, one end to the other, her slicing motion sure and quick.

I hadn't called, just dropped by in the middle of the afternoon.

"Auntie Irma doesn't think they should send Grandma home," Mom was saying.

"She isn't well enough?" I asked. "Or doesn't Grandpa take proper care of her?"

"He can't anymore. But he thinks he can. He's being very stubborn."

While my grandmother was in the hospital, my grandfather had put water on to boil and left the kettle on the burner until the kettle boiled dry and the metal glowed red. He wasn't allowed to drive but would forget, and pace, furious that he couldn't find his keys.

"It's hard to know if I should go. I was there two weeks ago."

Today might not be the day to tell her. She already had so much on her mind. But I felt an inner urgency. I needed to talk with her soon. Because I thought she might already know. Last week when I'd come for dinner she'd handed me a newspaper article about a pastor who'd confessed his attraction to men.

"I don't know why he'd want to make that public," she said.

I sat at the table with my head bowed, reading. I knew she was waiting for me to say something. My face felt hot. I needed to pee.

"He seems pretty clear about where he's at," I said finally, lifting my head.

"Clear? How could he be? He's confused."

"Well, according to him, he was confused for a long time, and now he's clear."

"Homosexuals can be healed you know."

Mom scooped handfuls of chopped cabbage into the pot, then the carrots. She talked through the ingredient list out loud to make sure she hadn't forgotten anything. Soon the house would fill with the smell of simmering borscht and freshly baked bread.

If I was going to tell her, she would need to slow down enough to look at me, preferably sit. At that moment I was content to watch her stir the soup, adjust the heat of the element, check the bread.

If I was going to tell her today, then these would be our final moments of easy conversation, the final minutes where she didn't think I was going to hell.

It was in this kitchen not that long ago when she had said, as she held a scraper in one hand and a bowl of icing in the other, "If child molestation is the worst sin, and I think it is, then homosexuality comes a close second."

As soon as I said what I had come to say, we would step over an invisible line.

Mom, Dad, and Coralee arrived as I was opening a bottle of water for Cec. The three of them filled the doorway. Mom had her arms hugged across her middle. Cor, my youngest sister, married to Jeremy and eight months pregnant, was the only one of my siblings who lived in Calgary. Dad brought up the rear.

I was glad to see them—a reprieve from my solitary vigil. I never knew how Cec would react. She could be gracious and charming, or prickly and intractable. When we were with my family she would generally engage with good humour, and then the minute they were out of earshot she'd let loose her criticisms. "It's always chaos." "There's no plan." "Your mom never sits down."

Mom touched Cec's arm. "How are you doing? Are you getting good care?"

"The nurses have been great. They're giving me good drugs."

"I didn't realize the last time we saw you that you were in so much pain."

Two weeks earlier, middle of February, Cec had invited Mom and Dad, Cor and Jer, and their two boys, Aiden, 6, and Jonah, 4, to Dalton's Restaurant at the Greenwood Inn for a birthday dinner, my thirty-ninth. The Greenwood has a swimming pool and the boys had brought their swimsuits.

"I wanted you to enjoy yourselves. It was Lyn's birthday."

Cec had been moving slowly that night. When it was time to go to the buffet she'd leaned against me and whispered, "I feel like I'm going to pass out."

"Do you want to go up to the room?"

No, she shook her head, and took hold of my arm, gripped tightly. We walked slowly. I helped her put food on her plate. She hardly ate, smiled with effort. I don't remember what she said, what anyone said, or why we laughed. I was too aware of her hunched shoulders, the squint of pain.

Dad sat perched on the edge of one of the visitors' chairs. He looked sad, I thought, to see Cec vulnerable like this, and tethered to an IV. Over the last couple of summers Cec had become his golfing buddy. She would call him when she had a couple of free hours and they'd play nine holes, usually Harvest Hills, the two of them muttering about club selection, distance to the hole, how much that putt would break.

They had friendly debates about Bush politics and Liberal government excesses. They talked weather, farming, Cec's latest shipment of pipe to Kazakhstan, war economics, the threat of terror. Dad had probably talked with Cec more than anyone else in my family. He'd say to me, rhetorically, "I can't figure out how she gets her ball to go straight—the way she dips her shoulder like that." He'd shake his head, smiling to himself.

I can see, as clearly as though I'm there, the Harvest Hills Golf Course. Blue sky. Hint of breeze. Sun directly in my eyes. Cec is beside me.

She has been dead for several months, but inside my daydream she is entirely alive and turning away as I step up to the tee.

"Your swing is terrible," she says. "I can't watch."

I don't know what her problem is. My drives have been landing on the fairway, second shots flying straight.

The sixth hole at Harvest Hills allows me to hit my driver full swing. If I connect, my ball will land at the perfect place for me to take my second shot right at the green, over two sand traps. If my ball slices, I'll land in sand.

My driver feels light as I take a practice swing, hips squared to the ball, knees slightly bent. I imagine Tiger Woods at the top of his swing, the way he unwinds with full torque. I'm no Tiger Woods, but I know the arc of a good swing, and the sweet smack of connection.

My ball sails almost straight, a little left but lands on the fairway. Not bad. A decent lie for my second shot.

"You moved your hips!"

"Did not! Look where it landed."

"If you'd kept your hips still it would have gone further."

She's wrong, but I don't bother arguing.

I wait for her to hit. Her tee shots are usually straight but not very long. I think it bugs her that I'm hitting my tee shots farther than hers.

We walk toward our balls, me slightly ahead, pulling

our golf carts. I stop and wait as she hits her ball. It heads in the direction of the green but lands well short. I know this irks her. When I get to my ball, she is right beside me, watching as I calculate distance. Should I use a five iron? Maybe a six. The breeze is behind me. I think I'd prefer the five. Nice easy swing. Don't overpower it.

"Which club?" she asks.

"Five."

"Will that get you there? You might want to go with a four."

"Five should be good."

"A four would put you on the green."

My shoulders tighten, but I don't say anything. I take a practice swing. Feels like I'm swinging a tree stump. Why can't she hold her tongue? I wonder for a split second whether I should use a four-iron instead of a five. In that moment of hesitation all her criticisms over all the years come crashing in, and I know with a certainty that makes my hands grip the club like an axe that I don't deserve this. I never have. I'm not a lousy golfer, or an awful gardener. I'm not lazy. Or illogical, thoughtless, selfish. I don't deserve, and shouldn't have to listen to, one more unkind word.

In my daydream, I step back from my ball and say to her, "I'm finished!" As I say those words I feel the weight of their meaning. They carry all the strength that is in me. I've had long conversations with myself, inside my head, about why I am staying when I am miserable, why I don't leave. Saying the words, finally, in this dream—the words I never said to her directly—feels like an accomplishment.

Before she can reply I say, "I'm not listening to you anymore. You can keep talking but I'm done. After this round I'm not coming home." I give her one of those I-mean-business looks over the top rim of my glasses.

She opens her mouth to reply, but I turn my back to her. I step up to my ball, square my feet, draw my five-iron back, and release smoothly.

The ball sails straight, lands just short of the green.

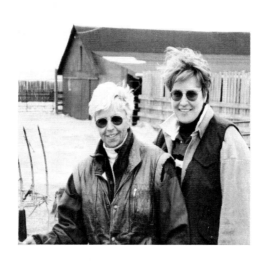

"I'd never kissed a woman before."

Day two of interminable tests. They rolled her down to the lab in a wheelchair, then again for a CT scan, then an X-ray.

The young doctor, Somers, from Emergency kept reappearing. Other doctors arrived, sometimes with a group of note-taking initiates. There was always a doctor in charge referring to a clipboard.

When the room was empty I would sit in an uncomfortable visitors' chair, my knees bent, feet resting on the metal rail of Cec's bed. The quiet of the room, the murmur of voices from the hallway sustained me like a heartbeat, faint but steady. Out the hospital window, a ceiling of high cloud, a film that filtered the light, made the whole room look wedding-photo soft.

I'd stopped asking Cec how she was doing. It irritated her to have to admit her pain. Instead I would ask whether the lab tech had been any good that morning, whether she'd thrown up during the night. It seemed as though she didn't throw up when I wasn't there. Or maybe she just wouldn't admit that she had.

Sometimes she'd lift her head and say, "Ice?" That was my cue to pick up an empty plastic cup from her table or get a new one from beside the microwave. I'd pass the nurses' station on my way to the ice dispenser near the main door to the ward—some of the nurses looked familiar—and someone would nod, smile.

When I was in her room I'd get restless. I needed to

move, anxious to leave. She could sense my agitation and it rattled her. So I'd leave. But I wouldn't be gone long before I'd feel an urgency to get back. Fear propelled me, a constant dread that something bad was about to happen. I didn't want to be there when it happened. And I didn't want to not be there.

I'd come back into her room as quietly as I could and settle back into one of the visitors' chairs, watch the quiet flush of her cheeks, her shallow breaths, in…and out.

I'd lean back, close my eyes, and try to figure out how many days I could take off work.

Cec motioned for me to pull my chair up closer. She reached for my hand and closed her eyes again. I sat watching her sleep and wondering at the small turns, the seemingly insignificant moments that shape the course of a life.

What if we had never met? What if I had been two minutes later for our meeting that day?

A shipping invoice we'd received was more than we'd been quoted. Tom had given it to me and asked me to get it fixed. I'd called the freight forwarding company and had been passed along to Cecile Kaysoe, the new general manager. She said that she would prefer to come to our office. She wanted to acquaint herself with our products and shipping requirements. We could review the invoice together.

I forgot about the meeting, hadn't dressed for it, hadn't booked the boardroom. I didn't remember until I saw someone with white-blonde hair standing in front of the reception desk and Euphemia waving at me. *Shit!* No choice now but to open the door to reception and say, "Sorry I'm late."

She had nodded, her grey eyes appraising as she shook my hand, a firm grip, "I was beginning to think you'd forgotten."

"It's been one of those mornings." My face got hot.

Months later as we lay in bed, still breathing hard after lovemaking, Cec said that she'd been about a minute and a half away from walking out the door that day.

"If I'd left, I would never have come back."

What if she had left? I wondered as I sat in one of the chairs at the foot of her bed. *What if she'd left and we'd never met?*

I remember being impressed that she wasn't overdressed— a pair of khakis with lots of pockets, a turtleneck, and a vest. She seemed to have anticipated the cement floors, the whirring machinery, the sawdust.

I opened the door to the manufacturing floor. I wasn't planning to give her a full tour, but we had to walk through the shop to get to the "bullpen," the cement-walled, high-ceilinged room where the sales team worked alongside the design engineers.

She touched my arm. "What is it you make here?"

"Consoles, for control centres."

"Out of wood?"

"The frames are metal." I bent so I could talk directly into her ear and not have to shout. "The exterior panels are made of wood and covered with laminate or veneer. Would you like to see?"

She nodded. I offered her a pair of ear protectors but she waved them away. "I have a table saw at home."

She did? I studied her again with a new appreciation as I led her to a console frame waiting to be outfitted with panels.

Was that the moment when I felt the first faint flush of attraction? Looking back now, I wonder. I know I was surprised, pleasantly, at her genuine interest.

"The frames are made of steel," I said, pointing, "with metal trays for the CPUs. Those are cable trays."

"Is that cherry veneer?" She ran her fingers along the wood grain on a stack of panels.

I was impressed that she could see the difference between real veneer and a wood grain laminate. "I'm not sure whether it's cherry—"

"I think it is." She surveyed the shop floor. It was clear she wanted a tour of the whole place, but we had the invoice to deal with and our conversation had already settled into friendly, almost familiar. I couldn't allow her to disarm me any further.

"The office is right over here." I led her away from the whine of the table saws into the open office area, rolled a chair from the side of the room to the space in front of my desk and motioned for her to take a seat. Five other desks ringed the room, no partitions. The engineers sat working quietly at their computers, listening to our every word.

Her chair tipped forward slightly as she lowered herself to sit. She quickly found her balance.

"So," she said as she leaned back carefully, "tell me what happened."

Her calm was unnerving.

She studied me with a contemplative look I couldn't decipher as I recounted my communications with her staff. *Did she know? In those moments? Did she have an inkling?*

She said, "Could I get a copy of your documents?"

"Sure."

"I'd like to review the file and get back to you." Her eyes were unsmiling but not unfriendly.

"That will be fine."

I hadn't given in, but at some level I felt as though I had.

Nell drummed her fingers on Cec's hospital room door even though it stood wide open.

"Hey?" Nell's soft, round face was a question mark. "I hope it's okay we came? Sarah really wanted to see you. We won't stay long." Nell walked softly into the room, as though still uncertain of her welcome.

Nell was married to Cec's brother Dennis, and it was highly unlikely that Dennis, gruff and funny and awkward around illness, would come to visit.

Four of Cec's eight remaining siblings (two had died within the last three years) lived in the city. The rest were scattered around the globe, in Vancouver, Germany, Long Island. Cec kept up a sporadic communication with each of them but often declined invitations to family get-togethers. She knew that in a pack her siblings could overwhelm. They were articulate and opinionated, and there always existed an equal potential for hysterical fun and biting sarcasm. Often sarcasm was the fun.

Sarah, Cec's niece, trailed behind her mom in the eyes-down slouch of a preteen who hates being taller than the boys.

"Come on in. Don't be shy." Cec waved them into the room.

Nell gave me a hug, kissed Cec on the cheek and handed her a bunch of daisies wrapped in cellophane.

She'd come straight from her shift at Brewster's, she said, and picked up Sarah at home. They'd stopped for a burger at Peters' Drive-In.

Sarah slumped into a chair, hands shoved into the pockets of her hoodie.

"How are you feeling?" Nell had pulled up a chair. She was goodhearted farm stock.

"All right for an old girl. Not a lot of fun when the parts give out."

"Have they said anything?"

Cec shook her head. "Not yet. They're doing a small exploratory surgery tomorrow to try to figure it out. May need a hysterectomy."

"We won't stay long. Sarah has to be up for school in the morning."

"Stay." Cec motioned for Nell to sit. "Lyn and I are getting sick of each other. She tries, but she makes a lousy nurse."

Nell and Sarah looked at me.

Cec was right. It's not that I wasn't willing to run for clean towels, fetch hot water for tea, help her into her housecoat. I just didn't know how to move in that slipper-footed, reassuring way. I was constantly jumping up, lunging instead of reaching. My movements startled. I said the wrong words at the wrong time.

"You get what you pay for," I said, and I got up out of my chair. I left the room.

Maybe that was rude, but I didn't care. Cec could say whatever she wanted to Nell about my inadequacies. I didn't need to hear it.

As soon as the hostess had seated us, Cecile took a lighter out of her purse, and a pack of cigarettes. Winstons. Unfiltered.

The hostess had asked whether we wanted to sit in smoking or non-smoking. I'd been just about to say, "non-smoking" when I heard Cecile say, "smoking."

Smoking? I didn't know she smoked. She hadn't asked me whether I minded. *Did I mind?* She didn't take her eyes off me as she lit up.

She had revised the invoice and called to say she'd bring it by in person, which she had, without warning, one warm Friday afternoon. I'd invited her to follow me into Tom's office. He'd already left for the weekend and didn't mind me using his office for meetings. His office window stood open. The breeze was gentle.

I watched her take in the deep-red walls of his small office, the large mahogany desk. The desk took up almost the whole room. There was just enough space for two chairs. I took the seat behind the desk.

She said, "Whose office?"

"Tom's. He's the owner. His father started the business. Now Tom is taking over."

"And the red walls?"

"Marking his territory, so to speak."

She smiled. "Is he going to keep the desk?"

"I don't know. He keeps changing his mind."

"I like the red. But the desk crowds the space." She was perched on the edge of the visitors' chair and turned to take in the room. She had on a cream golf shirt and a lighter vest. In the relative darkness of Tom's office, her hair looked shockingly blonde. White. Very Scandinavian. Which was probably the point. Not likely that was her natural hair colour.

I heard myself saying, "You look Scandinavian."

"It's the hair."

"Suits you. Is Kaysoe a Scandinavian name?"

"My husband was a Dane. His family name was Christensen originally, but everyone there is named Christensen so his great-grandfather or great-great-grandfather changed the family name to Kajsø (anglicized to Kaysoe).

"Your husband was a Dane?"

"He still is. He's just not my husband anymore."

"You've been to Denmark?"

"Lived there for twelve years."

"*Så du ka' godt snak Dansk.*" I couldn't resist.

"*Og det ka' du også.*" Her eyes opened in surprise. "*Er du Dansker?*" Her Danish had the sing-song lilt of an English accent. Danish is tonally very flat.

I switched back to English. "No, I'm not Danish." It had been a few years since I had spoken Danish and I wasn't sure how far I would get in a full-on conversation. "I lived there for a couple of years."

"*På Jylland?*" She was asking whether I'd lived on the Jutland Peninsula.

"You can hear it?"

She nodded.

"I'm going back for a visit this summer," I said.

"Oh, I'm jealous. Where will you be?"

"Visiting friends in Copenhagen, Odense, Mariager. Hoping to spend a couple of days in Skagen."

We talked our way through Copenhagen and up the Jutland Peninsula, the beaches at Skagen. Small as Denmark is, we didn't know anyone in common. Not entirely surprising, since I'd spent my time around Pentecostal churchgoers. She'd been immersed in the business world, based out of Copenhagen.

Suddenly she had to go. She had another appointment. Our goodbye was abrupt and hurried.

A few days later, a card arrived for me at work. I didn't yet recognize her handwriting, but I had a sense who the card was from as soon as I saw it. She'd sent a thank-you for the shop tour and a note asking whether I would like to meet for coffee.

I called her the next day. Her voice resonated at the lowest end of the female vocal spectrum. She filled her pauses between phrases with "ers" from deep in her throat. I had to press my ear to the receiver to hear her.

We agreed on an early dinner.

Across from me in the restaurant she leaned back, took a drag, and held her cigarette off to the side as though she wasn't actually holding it. She blew the smoke out the side of her mouth, a half-smile at the corner of her lips. Was she flirting with me? (Did I want her to be flirting with me?) She asked whether I wanted to order a platter to share, mostly deep-fried finger food. Not my first choice, but I nodded, "Okay."

She was saying something about freight forwarding but her words weren't registering. My eyes followed her fingers as she picked up a deep-fried zucchini, dipped it into the ranch dressing. Her fingernails were filed, the tips evenly rounded, coated in clear polish. She'd lived in Europe mostly. Also South Africa. She wasn't fluent in Afrikaans but she could get by. She was better in Norwegian and Swedish, also French, German, Spanish. She wasn't bragging, just stating, as Europeans do. She appeared entirely relaxed and intensely engaged at the same time. As soon as she stubbed out one cigarette, she lit another.

Months later, at our dining table, I watched as she sat with her head bowed, nail file in hand. She always filed.

Never clipped. She thought nail clippers barbaric, an indication of "lowbrow tendencies." My eyes followed her smooth strokes, from the bottom up, rounding at the top. Her hand was steady as she smoothed on a clear coat of lacquer. Always a clear coat, never colour. She blew on her finger, inspected the tip. A nail shaped to beckon, to catch hold of the wandering eye.

It was her quiet confidence that drew me to her. Her certainty. The way she made eye contact. She was comfortable in her body, at home in first class, accustomed to concierge service. But there was a weatheredness about her too. Fine lines fanned out around her eyes.

I could imagine her resting her elbows on her managerial desk, folding her fingers together. She knew how to place her hands lightly, deliberately, on top of a closed file folder.

Lawrence was Asian, which I hadn't expected. He moved with a matter-of-fact, flat-footed shuffle.

"On a scale of one to ten?" he asked as he took Cec's blood pressure.

"A three, or four. How much am I getting? Five?"

Lawrence checked her IV and nodded. "Is that enough?"

"I want to go down, to 2.5."

"Are you sure?"

"It's like I'm not in my body."

"You should be happy. People pay big bucks for that."

I knew Cec wouldn't like feeling disconnected. She loved to be hauling, pitching, lifting, sawing, nailing, digging, planting. Her other concern might have been with what she referred to as her "addictive personality."

"Just look at my family," she'd said as part of her explanation for why she never touched alcohol. "Most of them are addicts in one way or another. I should never have smoked that first cigarette. I didn't start smoking till I was twenty." She tapped her head as if to say, *not very smart.*

Lawrence pressed buttons on the IV machine. "Okay, 2.5 it is, but tell me if you need more."

A lab tech appeared in the doorway, white plastic case in hand, to collect pre-op blood.

Lawrence returned as soon as the lab tech was gone. He had a list of instructions. No more food. No water after eight o'clock. A porter would come for her at eight the next morning. He needed to ask her some questions. Some of these might seem redundant but this was part of surgery prep and he had to ask them all. He began with questions about allergies. Did she have a pacemaker? No. Any metal implants? No.

"Do you wear a hearing aid?"

No.

"Dentures?"

Yes, she nodded.

"Partial, or full."

"Full, top and bottom."

"They'll have to be taken out." He made a note.

I'd never seen her without her teeth, in our almost nine years together, not once. I could tell when she had taken her teeth out to soak them because she'd lock the bathroom door. I suddenly wondered whether it was a relief for her when she travelled and could leave her teeth out to soak at night.

"Have you ever had a local anaesthetic?"

"Yes."

"Any negative reaction?"

"No."

"General anaesthetic?"

"Once."

"Surgery?"

"D&C. After a miscarriage."

"When was that?"

"Uh, 1980-something. Eighty-two."

Cec had been certain it was a boy even though it was too early to tell.

"Another miscarriage in '84," she said, without prompting, which surprised me. She wasn't usually this forthcoming.

The second miscarriage at five months. A girl. Cec had named her Kate. Losing her babies had made her very sad. She had wanted children and said she still thought of them, imagined who they might have become.

Lawrence took the forms away. One of the residents would come by later, he said, to explain the surgery. "It's really more like a minor procedure, but there are always risks."

Wednesday, March 2

I almost made it to her room before they took her to the O.R.

I had promised that I wouldn't, so I'd had a debate with myself, and I'd hesitated, just long enough. When I arrived, breathless, at 8:02, she was gone.

"Taken down," the nurse said. She thought I could go down to the second floor, to the O.R. prep, and they'd probably let me see her.

But Cec had said she didn't want me to come so I stayed standing in the silence of her room, looking at the shiny bare lino formerly occupied by her bed. I felt oddly vacant and a little queasy. Her slippers were on the floor and beside them a pink basin. Both had been under her bed until she was rolled away. I walked to the centre of the empty room surprised by the fierceness with which I wanted her to come back.

It would be one thing for me to leave, another entirely for her to be taken away.

I left the ward, went down the elevator, and paced the long hallway from the main entrance to the flower shop and back again. I couldn't bear the idea of sitting in her empty room staring at the walls.

I got a coffee and sat in the coffee shop for a while.

I called Mom. No, she shouldn't come.

I went back up around eleven to check. She still wasn't there. I wandered to the visitors' room and stood, arms crossed, staring out a window, thinking about how surgery is like flying. Once the plane starts taxiing toward the runway, there is no turning back. They put you under. They cut you open. Anything can happen.

I tried to keep focused on positive thoughts, but I kept seeing the farmyard in the dark, the shadowy movement of cows in the corral, and Cec under the dim yardlight with a gun. Predators lurked in the night. Coyotes. Badgers. Porcupines. We lived under a constant threat of physical danger.

Like that night when the dogs all started barking at once—a holy ruckus. I'd bolted upright from a dead sleep. Cec was already out of bed and pulling on her clothes. "I'll go see what it is. You go back to sleep."

Several minutes later I heard a shot. Then smelled skunk. I scrambled out of bed. Cec was in the kitchen loading bullets into the clip.

"One shot and I ran out." She headed outside again. Another shot. And another. The smell of skunk grew chokingly thick. I stood on the back porch and waited for her to emerge from the shadows.

"It was a big one," she said. "Can you smell it?"

"Oh yeah, I can smell it."

She'd seen a flash of white under one of the cars. She knelt down and checked under each vehicle. Nothing. She heard a noise behind her and turned. The skunk was at the back door eating out of the dogs' food dish.

She took a few steps toward the skunk. The dogs seemed to know to stay behind her. She fired when she was ten feet away and hit her target, but one shot wasn't enough.

"I was out of bullets! By the time I got back out there, he'd gone about twenty feet, into the backyard, not far from the bedroom window. I had to put another half-dozen shots into him. This thing is useless!"

The bigger problem was how to dispose of a rather large, dead skunk.

"If I bury him, the dogs will dig him up."

The next morning she somehow managed to roll him into a garbage bag without actually touching him. She lifted the garbage bag into a plastic five-gallon pail and put the pail in the back of her company vehicle—"I wasn't going to use one of *our* cars!"—then drove down a back road where she offloaded him, pail and all, into the long grasses of a wide ditch.

We were sucking the liquid stench of skunk for days.

I paced the hall. I circled back to her room.

Routine, I kept telling myself, *barely an incursion*. She was tough. And she'd had anaesthetic before, so that shouldn't be an issue. The bigger question was how I had come to find myself here, pacing, worrying. Just weeks ago, I'd been contemplating my exit and now here I was, tethered to her hospital bedside, anxiously waiting to see what would happen next.

A few days after my first "date" with Cecile, our dinner of deep-fried (*Was that a date?* I'd wondered at the time but wasn't sure), she invited me over for a Danish dinner.

"In honour of your trip to Denmark," she said. "Do you like *frække deller*?"

"I love *frække deller*!" A classic Danish dish, oblong meatballs made of ground pork and veal.

"And *rød kål*?"

"And *rød kål*!" Pickled red cabbage.

She lived in Inglewood, an up-and-coming, shabby-chic community on the edge of Calgary's downtown.

"Turn right on 9 Ave," she said. "Then left as soon as you've passed Lou's Auto Body."

I pulled up in front of Cec's half-duplex on a breathlessly

hot summer day under a cloudless sky. She must have heard the car because she came wandering onto the front lawn as I turned off the ignition. She was wearing a black-and-white bikini and holding the end of a garden hose.

I stayed sitting for a moment, my eyes following her. I hadn't seen this much of her body at one time before. The hose was on and she was watering two small cedars that looked like they'd just been planted. Her skin hung loose on her bones, sagging under her biceps, folding over the waist of her swimsuit bottoms. What held me in my seat for an elongated moment, even after I'd pushed the car door open, were the folds of skin on her thighs. Her calves were firm, but the skin at her thighs hung like curtains. Too many cigarettes for too many years, I thought. Skin loses its elasticity.

Cec set the garden hose down and walked toward me with a slight swing in her hips. For the space of one deep breath, I fought off the urge to close the car door. I hadn't expected this—this hesitation.

I got out of the car. I raised my eyebrows. I gave her the smile I knew she was hoping for. I followed her into the house.

Days later, or maybe weeks, she said to me, stretching her nyloned calf from under a black skirt, "I have lovely legs."

"Yes," I murmured, "you do."

I was thinking to myself: *You have lovely calves. Lovely calves.*

I don't know whether Cec had any early inkling that she might be attracted to women. She said that she had wondered sometimes, but her questions had been fleeting and no opportunity had presented itself.

The possibility that I might be attracted to women wasn't

a consideration for me, not even the faintest possibility, until Denmark. And Anna. The only homosexuals I'd come across were in the bible, in Romans 2, Paul's rant about unnatural desires. Homosexuals were deviants. I imagined them as primarily homeless, aimless, miserable in their depraved despair.

Lying beside Anna, listening to her shallow breaths, enveloped in the sweet physical ache of her close proximity, was a revelation. But I couldn't shut off the voice of my Mennonite indoctrination, the one that said being with a woman was "unnatural." Or the anxiety at what this might mean. Because of what I now knew I wanted.

How deep does my religious programming reach? I wondered on those nights when I lay as close to Anna as I could without actually touching.

I'd sat through sermons on jealousy, greed, covetousness, idolatry, lasciviousness, licentiousness, concupiscence. I knew all about the dangers of temptation, the damnations of desire. I'd done my level best to stay away from sins that could get me into eternal trouble.

Did I have some kind of genetic predisposition to obeying rules? Maybe not all the rules (I consistently resisted putting on a dress) but certainly the big ones. That might sound crazy, but it felt possible.

Regardless of my Mennonite lineage and conservative Christian upbringing, an undeniable realization continued to grow: I was attracted to Anna. I wanted to be with a woman.

It's not that I found men unattractive, but up close my interest eventually waned. Even with Danny Reardon, and he was a great kisser, surprisingly soft lips.

I've thought about Danny often through the years, even though I haven't seen him or talked with him since our graduation from high school.

He was unruly, wild, and edgy with mischievous dark

eyes, a long, slow grin. He hadn't cared much for school or schedules or being pinned down to anything. Danny had his own relationship to the concept of time and could attach sexual innuendo to any word. His talk was often suggestive, never explicit, and always in a laughing way that wasn't invasive. He flitted in and out of my line of vision, never demanding, physically uninhibited.

When Danny kissed me, I realized that Brent was a lousy kisser. I'd "gone out" with Brent for all of about three weeks and had been tempted to tell him that he should take kissing lessons from Danny, but I'd bit my tongue. Danny and I weren't "going out." We had this understanding, never articulated, that there were no rules for him, or me, or "us." We could go anywhere, do anything, with anyone. No need to report in. No jealousy. None. In either direction.

Danny would often drive me home across the unending flatness of Manitoba prairie in the wee hours of the morning. He'd park the car under my parents' bedroom window and shut off the engine. I was afraid my parents might wake up. Danny didn't care. His large, warm hands pulled my shirt out of my jeans and found my belly, then my breasts. He seemed to know that I wouldn't let him past first base, or second, or wherever it was we were. He didn't push.

One night Danny and I drove to Winnipeg, about an hour north, to see a movie, just the two of us. That didn't happen very often. Usually there were others.

On the way home, he took my hand and sent me a kind of Morse code, a rhythmic insistence. We stopped talking. It felt as though he was reaching into my body. My heartbeat quickened. He held on tighter.

When we got to his place he kissed me. His easy languidness was gone. He pulled me on top of him, as much as the car would allow. He had an erection. He was undoing his jeans.

I pulled back.

"Please," he said. The only time he'd ever asked. "Just your hand."

I wish I'd said yes. If I could wind back the clock to any event in my life, I'd go back to that moment. But I was thoroughly inexperienced and I'd been warned about the way that boys reached "the point of no return" with lightning speed. There would be no turning back.

"I can't. I'm sorry."

My refusal wasn't just about sin and damnation. I wasn't overly keen on the male scent—a little too animal, sometimes overpowering. I wasn't partial to hairy chests or the bristly rub of facial hair. I held a mild curiosity about penises and their ability to inflate, but was content to leave them safely contained behind closed zippers.

Danny got out of the car, slammed the door, and zipped himself up with a shrug of frustration.

Cec's *frække deller* tasted authentically Danish. We cut them in half and laid them on rye bread, covered them with warmed *rød kål*, ate with our forks in our left hands.

"These are great! Or, should I say, '*Det smagt rigtig godt!*'"

"*Velbekom,*" she smiled.

We were sitting on wooden benches at a wooden table in a dining corner of her living area. The benches looked homemade. Either that or she'd found them at a garage sale.

"I made the landlord agree to put in new carpet before I signed the lease," she said.

I took a second *frække deller*, cut it in half, and laid the two pieces on another piece of dark rye bread, scooped pickled *rød kål* on top.

"And I had to paint the place. It was in bad shape."

"You did the painting yourself?"

She nodded. The exterior looked weathered and weary, but the inside was fresh and light.

"I hope you got a break in the rent."

"He paid for the paint and gave me the first month free."

"It's a big job to paint a whole place."

"I like painting. It's therapeutic. Like gardening."

"You have a garden?" Her skin was several shades darker than the first time we'd met, the bronze of someone who spent time in the sun. The dark brown of her skin created an even greater contrast with the white-blonde of her hair, which was close-cropped and spikey.

"The backyard was hard-packed dirt and weeds when I moved in. Looks like a jungle now."

"And you lived in South Africa?"

"My husband, at the time, was transferred there by his company."

"What did he do?

"Sold sailboats."

"And you?"

"Freight forwarding."

We both fell silent, chewing.

"How did you meet?" I was asking a lot of questions, personal ones, but she didn't seem to mind.

"Jens? My husband?"

I nodded.

"He was my boss, at the auto body shop where I worked."

"How old were you?"

"Eighteen."

"And what were you doing at the auto body shop?"

"Writing up estimates."

"You know cars?"

"Didn't know much then. I know more now."

"But how could you—I mean, don't you have to know a lot about cars to write estimates?"

She shrugged. "If you sound like you know what you're

talking about, people believe you, especially if you're a woman. Have you noticed? The way most women talk? With a rising intonation? Like they are looking for approval?"

I liked the sound of her voice, at the lower end of the female range except when she mimicked the questioning inflection. She was right. Women did that all the time and it made them sound subservient. I liked her facility with words, the way her mind worked.

"So you're a good bullshitter." I was grinning.

"It's an art form."

"I'll bet it is. Thanks for the warning."

"Most of my bullshit is more true than most people's truth." Her eyes were smiling. I could feel myself relaxing into an ease of communication and a sense of familiarity.

"Really!"

"Yes, really."

After she married Jens they moved to Victoria, lived there for a year, then moved to Denmark. They'd planned on staying in Denmark for a year, but one year had stretched into six. Cec completed an undergraduate degree at the University of Copenhagen and then apprenticed as a freight forwarder. When Jens was offered a job in Johannesburg they moved to South Africa. Cec got her masters there at the University of Johannesburg.

When she asked me how it was that I'd come to work at Hanson, I told her about my recent graduation from university with a degree without any practical application— a BA in Russian language and literature.

"Well," she said, with a head tilt and shrug of understanding, "my masters is in philosophy. Not exactly practical either."

I got the job at Hanson, I told her, because I'd gone to a friend's birthday party where I was introduced to Gwen, a friend of a friend. We'd sat on the back porch and talked for a couple of hours. Her husband was working at Hanson Consoles and they were looking for a proposals manager.

She gave me his phone number and said she'd tell him I would call.

As I sat for long hours at Cec's hospital bedside, I thought about the connections and the coincidences—*were they chance? or were they fate?*—that had to happen for us to meet.

What if I had decided not to go to the birthday party? What if I hadn't met Gwen or later called her husband about the job? Would I ever have met Cec? Or found myself sitting across from her eating her homemade Danish frække deller?

"*Tak for mad*," I said, the traditional Danish thanks after a meal.

"I'm glad you enjoyed it. I'll clear this later." Cec got up from the table and reached out her hand. "I'll show you my workshop." I thought for a second that she wanted me to take her hand but she turned and headed for the stairs, motioning me to follow.

The basement of her half-duplex was one large, unfinished room with a cement floor. In the centre was her workbench, two large pieces of plywood resting on sawhorses. On the makeshift work table: a hammer, power drill, Skil saw (although I didn't know what it was called at the time), nails, screws, shavings, chunks of wood. The floor was covered with a film of sawdust.

"What are you making?"

"A bench. This will be the seat." She held up two pieces of wood. "And these will be the legs." There were pencil markings on the wood. "I wish I had a router. It'd be easier."

I didn't ask what a router was. I was standing as close to her as I could without actually touching. I shoved my hands deeper into my pockets. I liked the way the spider lines at her eyes creased when she smiled. She pointed at the bench legs and I leaned closer, trying to decipher her scent, an oaky sweetness.

"I'd like to see the bench when it's finished."

"I'm going to build a picnic table next, for the backyard."

"Wish I knew how to use power tools." I picked up the hammer.

"I could teach you."

"Would you?"

"Sure. You can help me with the bench."

"But, I'm leaving for—"

"When you get back."

I set the hammer down. "Me and power tools…might be a dangerous combination."

"I'll make sure you don't hurt yourself." She touched my arm. "Would you like tea?"

"I would, but I have to get going. I still have a lot to do…to get ready…"

"Sure you can't stay a little longer?"

"I'm really sorry but I have to go."

"It's still early."

I couldn't tolerate this close proximity to her for much longer, but I didn't say that. I said that I couldn't stay but I would help her build a bench when I got back.

She said okay, I had to promise. She headed up the stairs. I was close on her heels, one step below her when she reached the landing.

"Send me a postcard?" She turned.

I nodded. She opened her arms. I opened my arms too, to give her a hug, and found myself kissing her. My knees threatened to give way. My lips parted to the probe of her tongue. I managed to remain upright. I was coming undone, but still coherent enough to know that I was living inside a cliché—the locking of lips followed by the ripping off of clothes. I'd watched this in movies and rolled my eyes. But there I was, barely able to hold myself upright, surprised at how instantly my body had responded, and with such abandon. I'd never capitulated like this before. But then, I'd never kissed a woman before. Only men. Well, actually, horny young males.

But when Cec kissed me, it was different. I was different. I didn't resist.

I let her lead me to the bedroom.

I shed my clothes.

I abandoned reason, something I had never let myself do with a man.

Cec's false teeth were chattering, her lips white and rimmed with blue.

"Relax, just relax," she instructed herself. She was shivering. They had rolled her back into her room, guardrails up. Her dentures were in place but her cheeks looked as though the air had been let out. She shuddered.

"Just relax," she whispered, eyes closed.

A nurse in a blue smock with white teddy bears came in to take Cec's pulse. "Would you like some morphine, dear?" in the singsong of a Newfie. Cec wouldn't have to open her eyes to know she liked this one.

A slight nod.

"And a blanket?"

"I'll get that." I knew where the blankets were, on the supply cart just outside the door. I unfolded one over her. "That should help." I touched her hand. Her skin was clammy.

"Have to…relax." She was trying to clench her teeth but they were chattering too hard. Her eyes opened, small slits.

"You're doing great, Babe." I tried to keep my voice steady, reassuring.

The nurse was back with a thermometer. "Can you hold this under your tongue, love?" She had wavy brown hair, a sturdy but huggable figure. "My name's Jessie." She put her hand reassuringly on Cec's shoulder. "A bit of fever's to be expected. Let's be sure this button works." She pushed the CALL button. A static voice said, "Hello?"

"It's okay, darling. Just testing." Jessie released the button. "If you need me, you push it," she said as she left.

Cec was still shivering. "Fever?"

"It's okay, Babe. You're okay."

"I'm okay," Cec said. She seemed to believe me. Her shaking had begun to subside. Jessie was back with a fresh bag of morphine.

"This'll help, and I'll bring an aspirin if you want it."

"I'm okay," Cec whispered.

"Yes, you are, Hon, you're doing great. You'll be up and giving me the gears in no time."

Cec's eyes closed. Her shivering stopped. Her mouth opened.

"It's like she stops breathing," I said to Jessie.

"Just for a few seconds. Morphine slows her mind. The pain doesn't get to her brain. That's what she needs right now."

Jessie left the room. I lowered a guardrail and pulled a chair up to the bed. My elbows on my knees, I rested my forehead in my hands. Her blue lips, her white cheeks, I couldn't not know anymore. *A serious health issue.* My eyes filled with tears, and I smeared them down my cheeks with the palms of my hands.

Soon they would have the lab results. Someone would say.

An orderly brought a lunch tray for Cec, an egg salad sandwich on brown and a bowl of watery vegetable soup.

"Am I allowed to eat?" She was sitting up, colour in her cheeks.

"Yes, I think so, the kitchen sent this. But wait, I'll ask." He disappeared and returned a couple minutes later. "Yes," he said, "it's fine."

Cec took a bite of sandwich, a few spoonfuls of soup, another bite of sandwich.

"How is it?"

"I'm not as hungry as I thought. You want the rest?"

"No thanks." The thought of swallowing made my stomach turn.

"Is there a dish?" Cec asked.

"A dish?"

"I think I'm going to throw up."

I found a pink plastic basin on the floor under her bed and handed it to Cec. She sat for a moment with her head bowed. Up came the egg, bits of bread, peas and carrots. I wasn't sure whether to move closer and put my arm around her or give her space. I perched on the edge of the bed, within arm's reach. She vomited again.

I filled a plastic cup with water but she waved it away.

"To rinse your mouth."

She took a small sip, swirled it around in her mouth and spat into the bowl.

"Is that it?"

She nodded, "I think so. Who said it was okay for me to eat?"

I took the basin from her, went into the bathroom, dumped the contents into the toilet, rinsed the bowl, dumped that into the toilet, flushed. I was surprised by my calm. The sound of retching usually made me queasy.

I set the basin under Cec's bed. "We'll keep this close."

She patted the bed beside her and I sat down.

"I'm so sorry."

I put my arm around her, gently. "It's okay. I usually don't do very well with bodily functions, but I'm okay. You don't need to apologize."

A few minutes later Cec said, "Dish! Get the dish."

Jessie came into the room as Cec was rinsing her mouth.

"Don't like egg salad?" Jessie took the basin from Cec. "Are you finished or is there more?"

"Oh, there's probably more." Cec cleared her throat. "But you can take it."

Jessie emptied the basin and brought back a clean one. "On your table so it's close?"

"No." Cec waved it away. "Don't want to look at it."

"I can get it for her if she needs it." I set the basin on the floor.

"Who said I could eat?"

"I don't know, but you probably shouldn't have." Jessie pulled on a pair of thin plastic gloves. "Let me have a little look at your dressings, okay, Hon?" She pulled the curtain closed around Cec's bed and said to me, "You don't need to stay."

"It's okay. I'm okay. If it doesn't matter to you—" I looked at Cec.

"She can stay."

Jessie pulled back Cec's blanket and lifted her nightie. Cec's stomach had ballooned. She looked six months pregnant. Her legs were thick, twice their normal girth. Jessie peeled back the clear tape that held the white gauze dressing in place.

"It's seeping quite a bit," she said. The incision was tiny, located a couple of inches to the right of Cec's belly button, about half a centimetre, no stitches, just a small slit oozing a clear fluid. The gauze was drenched. Jessie swabbed the area with an antiseptic cloth. Fluid continued to ooze.

"We'll have to try to keep up with this," Jessie said as she taped a new piece of gauze into place. "Let me know when this is soaked. I need to look at the other one too. Can you sit up?" She helped Cec lean forward, untied the back of her gown.

"Can you take your arm out?" Cec freed her right arm and lifted it up so Jessie could check the bandages.

A couple of weeks before I drove Cec to Emergency, she'd said, "Look at this." She'd leaned her head to the side so that I could get a clear view of the red, puffy lumps along the right side of her neck. Under her arm too, she said, just on the one side.

Cec had showed the doctor she went to see in Didsbury. He'd said that it was probably viral and prescribed an antibiotic. The lumps hadn't gone away.

Since she was already under, Cec's gynecologist had decided to biopsy the lumps under her arm. The incision was about an inch long, held together with stitches. It looked raw and crusted with blood.

I sat at the foot of the bed while Jessie cleaned the wound.

"Not very pretty, eh?" Cec said.

"There's a good reason I didn't become a nurse."

Dr. Kendrick was back again. She pressed on Cec's belly, "Any bowel movements?"

"Bowel movements aren't exactly my specialty. And who said I could eat?"

"Someone said you could eat?"

"The guy who brought lunch. I said that I didn't think I should eat right after surgery."

"It's best to wait until your bowels are functioning."

"I keep throwing up."

"We'll put you on liquids for a while. Give you some Boost."

Cec turned up her nose. "Geriatric food."

Kendrick lifted the white gown with the tiny blue flowers, held her stethoscope to Cec's belly. "Has anyone talked with you about the surgery?"

"No."

"The final lab results should be ready within the next couple of days, Friday at the latest," she said as she pulled Cec's nightie back down over her tummy, "but I can tell you that based on what we observed," her voice disarmingly friendly, "it's looking suspicious for cancer."

Cec turned to me. "There it is," she said, "the C-word."

She didn't seem surprised or upset. "But that's not for sure," she said to Kendrick.

"We won't be able to say with certainty until we get the lab report."

"Did they take the lump out?"

"He decided it would be best not to remove the mass. But he biopsied everything."

"If the news is bad," Cec turned to me, "we'll take that road trip we talked about. Sell the farm, buy an old school bus, drive across the country."

If the news is bad? I hoped she wasn't serious. "A school bus would be uncomfortable," I said, imagining her bumping along in the back.

"Or a van. We'll need room for the dogs."

"The dogs?"

"Well, Noddy."

"I think we should wait for the lab results before we—"

"You don't want to go!"

"I do want to go."

"Don't lie to me!"

"I mean it, Babe. We just don't know."

She squinted hard at me trying once again to discern my sincerity. I didn't blink. We'd often talked about a road trip. But she hadn't been in pain then.

"I'll be right back." I left her room, walking quickly, trying to outpace my tears and the image I couldn't shake of her thin body in a white gown on a rattling hospital bed, IV pouch swinging.

I kept my head down, eyes on the flecked tile. The visitors' room was empty. I dropped into a chair feeling light-headed and heavy at the same time.

C-word. Road trip. Sell the farm...the farm...the farm.

Griff and Charlie. I needed to check on them. They'd be hunting gophers, and lying on the deck. As long as they stayed in the yard and didn't wander. Especially on clear nights. Full moons. That was when the coyotes came out in force. The coyote pack would send a lone female in close to a farmyard, at the edge of gun range. She'd yelp as though she was in heat. Any dog that responded to the call would get himself ambushed by the rest of the pack. Griff had never fallen for that trick, not yet anyway. He'd sit next to Charlie on the deck, and the two of them would throw their heads back and howl in off-key harmony.

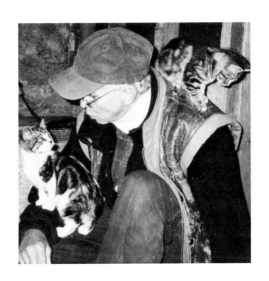

"We need a Plan B"

Thursday, March 3

At 6:03 a.m. I was jerked from the thin surface of sleep by the shrill jangle of my cellphone. PRIVATE CALL.

"Hello?"

Cec's voice, barely a whisper. "I haven't slept."

"But, I thought—"

"They brought me a new roommate. Middle of the night. Drug overdose. She hasn't shut up."

"Shit!"

"She keeps calling for the nurse. She wants a drink of water. Then she spills her water and wants a nurse to clean it up. Then she has to pee."

"I'm sorry, Babe." I was wide awake. Beside me, Noddy stretched.

"You need to get me out of this room!"

"I'm coming."

"Not *now*!"

"Why not?"

"It's too early."

"But I'm—"

"There's no point."

"Then why'd you call?"

"I need a different room."

"Okay, I'll get you a new room."

"It's the middle of the night."

"It's almost morning. I'll come."

"No, not now."

"Okay, I'll come later."

Silence at the other end of the line. Then a dial tone.

I flipped my phone shut, thumped my head back onto the pillow. There was no way I would fall asleep again. *Why had she called?*

I tiptoed into her room. She was in one of the visitors' chairs, her feet up on the bed, legs covered with a blanket, eyes closd.

I was about to tiptoe out again when a voice from the other side of the curtain said, "Edna, is that you?"

Cec rolled her eyes as she opened them. She said, "You shouldn't have come."

"But you called. You said."

"I said you shouldn't come."

My body tensed with the familiar hurt and fury at her impossibility.

"So you called me at six o'clock this morning because—"

"I need to sleep, Lyn."

"You need your own room." I considered walking out. But what would be the point? "Who's your nurse?"

"Lorraine."

From the other side of the curtain: "Is there a nurse? Edna? Is there a nurse?"

Cec took a deep breath. "I'm NOT Edna!"

A heartbeat of silence, then: "Nurse?"

"There is no nurse!"

Cec was right. I shouldn't have come.

Cec leaned back in her lawn chair, cigarette between her second and third fingers. We had gone out onto the deck so she could have her after-dinner smoke.

"So, why did you say no to Christian's engagement proposal?"

"I didn't say no. I said I had to think about it."

"But you didn't let him put the ring on your finger."

"That's not the same as saying no."

Cec had been seeing Christian for seven years. She was still seeing him when she'd begun her transition back to Canada. He was a Danish photojournalist, on the road more than he was home. He'd go to Bali on assignment and Cec would arrange a "business trip" to Bali, trek with him up into the mountains, to remote villages, wander the beaches. Sometimes she'd write an article to accompany his photos.

Christian got her a media pass into Sarajevo when it was under siege, she said. They'd hunkered down with the other journalists, dodged sniper fire.

She talked about him and her adventures matter-of-factly, no hint of trying to impress. She gave me no reason to question, though when I thought back later, dodging sniper fire did seem a bit extreme.

She watered his lawn when he was away, tossed out food remains that were turning black in his fridge. But she refused to do his laundry. Or cook for him. They'd eat in restaurants. She had the money. So did he.

"Why did you have to think about it?" I asked.

"He kept talking about how when we got married I'd

have to quit my job. My *job*?! I owned my own company! I didn't have a *job*!"

She told him that they'd talk when she got back from Vancouver. She was going to explore a potential real estate investment, a commercial development.

"I'll show you the property when we go," she said. "Right on the waterfront."

"We're going to Vancouver?"

"If you want to."

I wanted to. And we did, one long weekend. We stayed on Granville Island, explored the market and the artist studios, walked along the beach. Cec took me to her favorite antique shops and hole-in-the-wall restaurants. She had an uncanny ability for finding interesting out-of-the-way places.

She showed me where she had lived when she'd first moved to Vancouver from Denmark. And she showed me the commercial development property. It was a business tower on the waterfront with stores on the ground level.

Eventually she'd sold her freight forwarding company in Denmark and began spending more time in Vancouver. She rented an apartment, a "flat" as she called it.

"I'd always known that I'd move back to Canada, to be closer to my mother."

"What did Christian say when you moved?"

"I still had my house in Copenhagen."

"But did you tell him about—"

"It was just a place to stay."

She took a drag and stared off into space.

"Do you still have your house in Copenhagen?"

"No. I sold it. Had to."

I waited but she didn't seem inclined to offer up anything else.

Finally I said, "Had to?"

She exhaled a long trail of smoke as she said, "I lost my investment in the real estate deal." She stubbed out her cigarette, lit another. "You know how they say you should never put all your eggs in one basket? Well, it turns out they're right."

I waited.

"I had most of the money I needed for my share but I didn't have all of it. I called someone—don't ask who, it doesn't matter—and asked whether he wanted in with me. He said he'd wire me the money. But," she took a deep breath, "his money didn't arrive on time. I missed the deadline. Had to forfeit my investment."

"All of it?"

She nodded. "And pay a penalty."

"But it wasn't your fault!"

She shrugged. "My signature. My risk."

"You should sue the guy!"

"I shouldn't have tried to play with the big boys." She blew smoke out her nostrils. "Had to sell my house, my cars, everything. All I had left were a few boxes. They're still at Christian's, if he hasn't thrown them out."

"Does he think you're coming back?"

"I don't know what he thinks."

"But he must have called."

"He called." She tapped the ash from her cigarette into an ashtray.

"What did you tell him?"

She didn't respond.

"Does he still call?"

I thought she might be getting annoyed at all my questions, but then she said, "Not for a long time."

"Did you have second thoughts about moving?"

"About moving in with you?"

"About moving away from Denmark."

"If you're asking whether I'm having second thoughts about you, the answer is no."

That wasn't what I'd asked.

Cec motioned me closer. I bent down. She whispered, "I don't plan to hang around like this for very long."

I straightened, "What do you mean?" I knew exactly what she meant.

A part of me was hoping that I was wrong. Another part of me wanted to slow down the knowing.

"We need a Plan B." *Plan B   Plan B   Plan B* Her voice echoed through my mind. "You'll have to figure something out."

"But…I don't think…" *I couldn't. I'd never. I didn't have the faintest clue what to—how to—*

"I'm crazed with pain, Lyn, half out of my mind, and it's not going to get any better."

I steadied myself against the bed rail. She wasn't asking. She was instructing, confident in her executive ability to give an order and have it carried out.

"You get the stuff and we'll take care of it, just you and me," she said. "No one else needs to know."

"What stuff?" I'd never smoked a cigarette never mind tried to get a hold of anything heart-stopping. *And now she wanted me to*—I didn't even want to think my way through to the end of the thought.

"Whatever we need, you'll have to get it ready."
WE need?

"Lyn, please. There's no one else I can ask." Her voice was suddenly weak and, for the first time, pleading.

There was no one else she would ask. I was it. Without me, she couldn't. Well, maybe she still could.

And she still might. I had learned not to underestimate her.

A cleaning woman appeared in the doorway pushing a mop. Cec was waiting for me to nod or say something. I could feel tears rising. Furious tears. Helpless tears. I walked out of the room.

Did she really expect me to—? Shit! I wish she hadn't—How could she? Just like that.

There was a young couple in the visitors' room. The woman glanced at me, then away. I must have had a wild look in my eyes.

The stuff. What stuff?

I kept seeing her eyelids falling closed, dry lips parted, face ashen.

No one else needs to know.

No one else had ever known. It had always been just me. Solitary confinement. I was tired of never saying anything to anyone. But who would I talk to? If I said anything, even one word, I had this sense that the words would keep coming... and coming. If I said anything, I would say everything.

I sat down in the chair closest, leaned back and hugged my arms around myself. When I came to the end of my thoughts, the dead end of all the rationalizing, I knew without a doubt that I would fail her. There was no way I could make a decision that I could live with. Either way. I was damned.

I wanted to call Mom. But she'd hear the tears in my voice. And then I'd tell her.

Why wasn't there a form I could fill out, like the requisition for her TV? Or, better yet, a form *she* could fill out, an arrangement she could make, with someone whose job it was, who could explain the options. Someone who could get *the stuff.*

I should have packed my suitcase when I had the chance. Boxed up my books. Taken Noddy. Even though Cec would have been furious.

I'd given Noddy to her as a birthday present. We'd visited the breeder together and Cec had picked him out of the litter. He was the smallest, and the most inquisitive. When he was old enough to be weaned, Cec went to pick him up. What I hadn't anticipated was that Cec would insist Noddy sleep between our pillows.

"But what if we smother him?"

"We won't. Besides I'll need to take him out during the night. If he wriggles, I'll wake up."

When I tried to lean over him to give her a good-night kiss, she shielded him with her hand. "Careful!"

I rolled away. She'd been pulling back for months, saying she didn't want to lead me on, didn't want to raise my hopes. Her desire had dried up. Dead libido. Overnight it seemed. She wasn't sure why. It had nothing to do with me. I shouldn't take it personally. I wasn't sure how she thought it would be possible for me to not take it personally.

She'd thought about asking her doctor for one of those chemical aphrodisiacs, she said, but she didn't like to take drugs. Or maybe she should eat more oysters? She gave me an apologetic smile. Which made me want to say it was okay, give her a kiss. I wanted to tell her that kisses were enough. But I knew I'd be lying. And she'd know too.

My attempt at a good-night kiss was a test.

By setting Noddy between us she was admitting defeat. She failed the kiss test. She was failing me.

Sex had come undone. In some ways it felt as though it had stopped abruptly. But if I looked back, I could see that it had unravelled slowly, a soft thread of promise that had stretched out into a long, thin line I was no longer allowed to cross.

"Edna" persisted. I didn't know her name. She was stubborn and vocal. For a second night in a row Cec hadn't managed a minute of sleep.

I marched over to the nurses' station with my hands on my hips—determination fuelled by agitation. I'd never spoken with this nurse before, but that didn't matter. I told her, firmly, that it was absolutely necessary to move Cecile into a private room. We were prepared to pay.

The nurse leaned forward, undaunted by my agitation. I thought for a moment that she might reach out and put her hand on my arm.

I didn't think about it until later: She had seen Cec's chart. She knew the lab results. She understood what was coming.

"We have a room for her."

"You do?"

"As soon as it's been cleaned."

"A private room?"

She nodded. "You can go have a look. Number thirteen. At the end of the hall."

I walked back to Cec's room mildly triumphant, "You're getting a private room!"

Cec's face was flushed. The look in her eyes stopped me. I knew that look. Everything had shifted. I'd seen this happen before, like a switch had been flipped.

"That sweater is so bulky! Don't you have something else you can wear?"

"Did you hear me? You're getting your own room."

"Won't matter," she said.

"No more roommate. It'll be better."

"The doctors come…" She paused. "And the soup… nurse…" Her eyes closed and her head tipped back. Her mouth hung open.

I stood and waited for her to come back, my arms folded defensively, ready for her to pick up where she'd left off. One other time when she'd been on me about something, I'd said to her: "Why do you have to be so difficult?"

Her response was immediate: "You think *this* is difficult?!"

"The nurse…" she said as her head nodded forward again.

"You need the nurse?"

"No." She shook her head. She seemed disoriented but still annoyed.

"A new room will be quieter, Babe."

"Don't call me that! Not in public."

"But there's no one—"

"They can hear you." She gestured toward the open door. "And put on something else for god's sake!"

The sweater I was wearing was a dark red fleecy with a zip up the front. Cec had bought it for me. Yes, it was bulky. It had to be, to cover the heft of me. I knew it wasn't the sweater Cec was objecting to. It was my rounded face, my wide thighs, my growing bulk.

When I met Cec, I'd weighed 182 pounds, a relatively slender six-feet tall. Eight and a half years later, I was tipping the scale (behind a locked bathroom door, for my eyes only) at 238. When I stood naked in front of the mirror and looked at myself in profile, my stomach bulged. Varicose veins were spreading their red-blue tentacles across my thighs. No wonder Cec had wanted the lights out when we made love.

My first instinct was protest. These additional pounds were not my fault. Cec bought the groceries, did most of the cooking, all of the baking.

But I was the one who opened my mouth and ate the muffins, took a second piece of lemon-blueberry pie.

"You need to work out," Cec had said, more than once. "Find something you can do out here on a regular basis."

"I could move bales."

"That's my job."

"Cleaning out the corrals is a good workout."

"Once a week is not enough."

I was doing deep-water workouts on my lunch hours. But the rate at which I consumed Cec's pumpkin loaf and rice pudding still outpaced, by a long stretch, the calories I managed to burn in the pool.

"I have an idea!" I said to Cec one day. I thought it was the perfect solution. "I'll walk, or maybe even run, up and down the hill a couple of times a day!"

The land along the west side of our property dropped sharply down to the creek. Getting up that incline would be a good workout, get my heart rate up.

I wondered later whether there was any way I could have anticipated her response.

"That's pretty selfish!"

Selfish?

"That will only benefit you. We have a farm filled with animals that need exercise. At the very least you should put a halter on one of the horses and lead it around."

I stood dumbstruck at her response, and also surprised that she could still surprise me.

"When I move bales it helps everyone."

Help everyone? I didn't realize that was a prerequisite. Later I wished I'd said that. It wouldn't have been a brilliant comeback but it would have been something. Better than the blank look I gave her as I fought back tears. Cec was right: I needed a thicker skin.

"How do you know?" My mother said the words like a challenge, as though she was certain that there was no way I could give an acceptable answer.

We were at the dinner table. My dad was there too, keeping his head down, eating quickly. He seemed particularly uncomfortable. Ever since I'd come out to my mom she'd been mostly sad around me with little to say except in small angry bursts.

Mom set down her fork. "How do you know that you are attracted to women?"

Her question wasn't really about my attraction to women. What she wanted to know was how it could be possible that I wasn't attracted to men.

There was nothing I could say that would satisfy her.

"Well, Mom, how do you know that you're attracted to men?"

"I just know. I just am."

It hadn't been quite that simple for me. My socialization and indoctrination hadn't allowed me to acknowledge my attractions with a simple, straightforward knowing. It had taken some unraveling, some secret admitting, and whispered conversations. But now I knew. I knew like she knew.

"I know too, Mom. It's the same. I just know."

My mother stared at me blankly. "No," she said, "it's not the same."

When I had moments to myself—walking down the hall, fetching ice, hot water for tea, checking the nurses' schedule— my mind would keep going back to Plan B. I knew that Cec was serious, and I understood why.

When her pain ramped up, when it bore down, when it settled in, there was no relief. It was torture. Unrelenting. Even when she finally agreed to 7.5 milligrams, and then to 10, the maximum, she received little relief. She cried out. She squeezed my hand until I thought she might break my fingers. There was nothing I could do. My helplessness was excruciating.

I'd had no idea that this kind of pain existed. Or that narcotics could be so maddeningly ineffectual.

There were moments when I considered putting a pillow over her face, just grabbing one and doing it. But then I'd get up to close the door and by the time I came back, my resolve would have dissipated. Maybe she'd want some warning, I thought, some say as to when.

The best idea I'd come up with was antifreeze. I could put it in a Gatorade bottle. She could drink it right after she'd sucked on one of those blue Popsicles; a few more blue drips on her hospital nightie wouldn't raise any alarms. Except I wasn't sure that she'd be able to keep it down, and I didn't know what antifreeze would do in the body, how much it might hurt.

I still wanted Plan B to be a number I could call, a person on the end of the phone who would ask, with clinical proficiency, for the necessary information and arrange to meet. The voice would be a deep, reassuring bass. I'd recognize him when he strode down the hospital hallway, his gait relaxed and self-assured. He'd get straight down to business.

I'd be able to see that she wasn't afraid at all. Then her eyes would close.

I'd push the CALL button. A raspy voice would answer and I'd say: "She's not breathing!"

I'd hear the rapid steps of white nursing shoes down the hall.

I'd feel a hand on my shoulder.

A voice would say, "You can go now."

Lorraine came with the news just after lunch: Cec's room was ready.

"Okay, people, get me out of here!" Cec waved at Lora. She'd arrived not long after Mom.

Lora took the vases from the shelf. Mom helped Cec into her wheelchair and pushed her down the hall. I gathered the toiletries, threw out used cups, collected the Get Well cards, her shoes, and slippers.

Cec's new room was airy and light with a large window and her own little bathroom. She seemed pleased, sitting with her blankets smoothed around her, her attendants in the high-backed chairs. There was a hush of expectancy. I knew that Mom had come for the same reason that Lora had come—to hear what the doctor had to say about the lab results.

Lora asked Cec whether she wanted to sleep? Should they leave?

"No," Cec waved her down. "Stay."

"I'll be right back." I left Cec with her ladies-in-waiting and went to the nurses' station. I asked the nurse behind the desk whether she had seen Dr. Kendrick.

She hadn't.

"Do you have any idea when she will be coming by?

"Soon," she lied. "I'm sure she'll be by soon."

She didn't know. The nurses never knew.

Dr. Kendrick was wearing a light-blue blouse and navy pants. With her curly hair and her breezy smile, she looked like a mom model out of a Sears catalogue.

"And how are we this afternoon?"

Cec gave her a blank stare.

"And your pain? On a scale of one to—"

Cec held up four fingers. She was waiting expectantly. We all were—each of us in a visitor's chair, our eyes on Kendrick. Today was the day. She should have the lab report.

Kendrick skimmed a page on her clipboard. "Senokot, lactulose, Losec..." she said under her breath. "And no stool yet?"

Cec didn't say anthing.

Kendrick put her stethoscope to her ears. "I think it's time to try Fleet."

"What's that?"

"An enema. Stronger than lactulose. It can be taken orally. There are also suppositories." Cec looked as though she was drifting. Her breathing stopped. Her eyes rolled up into her head.

"She's stopped breathing!" Mom sounded alarmed.

"She comes back."

When Cec's eyes rolled forward again she had a scowl on her face. "Move that crater!" Or maybe it was, "Move that critter!" Her speech was slurred. "Don't stand there!" She frowned, and then seemed to realize where she was. "Oh," she said, looking around the room, mildly bewildered. "I meant the other guy."

"How often does this happen?" Kendrick asked.

"Don't like it," Cec said.

"Often enough that she wants to keep her morphine really low."

"Don't like creeping foggy."

"You mean 'feeling foggy'?" I didn't usually translate

when her words came out jumbled, but I wanted to be sure Kendrick understood.

Kendrick nodded. "The right level, or even the right drug, or combination of drugs, is different for each person. It can take a while to figure it out. The palliative team will be taking over your pain control. They're the pain specialists."

I sat up at the word palliative. Since when had Cec become palliative? Kendrick's cheerful demeanour hadn't darkened, not for a heartbeat.

"This will be my last day as your doctor. A new resident, Dr. Steader, will be taking over."

Palliative means terminal.

"He may come by later today to introduce himself, or Monday morning."

Kendrick hugged her clipboard to her chest.

Wait a second! "Are the lab results in?"

"Has no one discussed them with you?"

"No."

Kendrick consulted her clipboard again, even though I was pretty sure she didn't need to.

"Well, it's definitely cancer; a kind that often begins in the cervix. This is a cancer that creates a lot of fluid. That's why you're seeing discharge from the incision site."

Kendrick picked up a felt marker and drew on the whiteboard at the foot of Cec's bed. She sketched the almost-heart shape of a uterus and the "horns" of fallopian tubes with circles for ovaries on the ends.

"The cancer very likely began here," she said, placing a dot on the right ovary. She sounded like a teacher giving a first grade lesson. "But it could have started in the cervix." Another dot at the top of the uterus. She turned to look at us, to make sure we were following. I glanced at Cec. She was sitting with her hands folded in her lap, attentive and expressionless. I thought she looked waif-like, and vulnerable.

"It's called squamous cell carcinoma." Kendrick wrote "squamous" on the white board. "As for the stage we're at," her tone still pleasant, verging on cheerful, "the cancer is advanced and aggressive."

She put the cap back on the marker and picked up her clipboard. *That was it?* She was gathering herself to leave. It was Friday afternoon and she didn't want to be having this conversation.

"What stage are we at?" I asked.

"Four."

I leaned back in my chair. *Stage four.*

Stage three meant the cancer had metastasized. Stage four was the final outpost. For most cancers there was no stage five. I wondered whether Cec understood. She looked thoughtful, contemplative. Her demeanour didn't change as Kendrick talked.

"Stage four means that the cancer has spread beyond the original site," Kendrick continued evenly.

That's diplomatic, I thought. I didn't know much about the stages of cancer but I knew Stage four was bad news. And I was having difficulty comprehending Kendrick's emotional balance. How she could be so—unconcerned? So matter-of-fact.

"Most of the pain you're experiencing is because of the fluid that the cancer is creating. An appointment at the cancer centre is being scheduled for you. The oncologist will be able to tell you more."

"The cancer centre? She'll have to go there?" That was on the other side of the city.

"She'll have to go there."

"Isn't there an oncologist here?"

"It's best she see a gyne-oncologist."

"There isn't one here?"

Kendrick shook her head.

"But her gynecologist—he's not a gyne-oncologist?"

"No."

If it was so important that Cec see a gyne-oncologist then why hadn't she been referred to one sooner? Why hadn't a gyne-oncologist done her surgery?

"Can't an oncologist come here? She's in so much pain."

Cec was nodding.

Kendrick shook her head. "I don't think that will be possible." She tucked her clipboard under her arm. "One of the nurses will let you know when the appointment is."

"But…" I got out of my seat.

Cec waved her hand at me, motioning for me to sit: "At least now we know."

That was it? She wasn't going to ask any questions? I had a million questions:

How far had the cancer spread?

Would she receive treatment?

What was her prognosis?

I had imagined a scene, like on television, when the doctor comes in and gives the terminal diagnosis and then says, *You have three months* (or six months, or a year) *left to live.*

"Thank you," Cec said. She sounded genuinely grateful. I think she was. She had always said that the hardest part was not knowing.

Kendrick shook Cec's hand and left quickly, before anyone could ask another question.

I looked down so no one could see my eyes: *Palliative. Stage four.*

"Well, there we have it," Cec said softly. "The verdict."

"Now we know." Lora's voice was barely a whisper. She was struggling to keep her composure.

Were they really going to make her go across the city to see an oncologist?

I wanted to sue them, for incompetence, all of them. Her family doctor. That doctor in Didsbury that Cec had liked so much. Her gynecologist, who was *not* an oncologist.

But especially the Didsbury doctor. I imagined him fair-skinned with blond hair, in a pressed white shirt, grey dress pants, saying in a deep voice, "This should help…we all have a few aches and pains…"

I wouldn't bother with her family doctor. He was an old man living in a grey-haired purgatory. But the doctor in Didsbury—Cec had trusted him.

Mom was the last to leave. I offered to walk her out. I needed to escape Cec's room.

"Was that what you were expecting?" Mom asked as we waited for the elevator.

"After her surgery one of the doctors said it was looking suspicious for cancer."

"Oh yes, you told me that. I think I was hoping—"

"What I don't understand is how she could get all the way to Stage four."

"Do you think Cecile knows what that means?"

"I don't know."

As we neared the main exit, Mom slowed. "I've been thinking…" She stopped and I nudged her toward the wall so the people behind us could get past.

"I wasn't very welcoming to Cecile when I first met her."

"That was a long time ago, Mom."

"I know. But I've been thinking—I was wondering—do you think I should apologize? For how I was?"

Her question surprised me. My mother's relationship with Cec had become relaxed and friendly, if a little careful.

"I don't think that Cec needs you to apologize."

"No?"

"No."

"I just don't want to have a regret—that I had the chance."

"If you need to, then you should. Say whatever you need to say."

"I should, shouldn't I?"

"Yes, you should."

"Just like I thought..." Cec was talking on her cell. I stopped in the doorway. Maybe I should give her some privacy? "Ovarian...that's where the mass was but it could have started in the cervix...th-that's right...yes, the reproductive bits, like I thought..." Her voice was bright. I pushed the door open. "I don't know, they haven't said...an appointment at the cancer centre...yeah, it's spread, that's why I'm so bloated... mhmm...stage four."

Cec said "Stage four" like she might have said "the back nine."

A tall, lean man with dark skin pushed Cec's door open. It was after dinner, well past the time when doctors normally made rounds.

Dr. Rajesh Sanjay introduced himself with a small bow of his head. He was tall, willowy, fine-featured, and spoke with a slight British accent.

Cec looked sleepy but lucid, and sat up a little straighter when he introduced himself as a palliative doctor. I wondered at Cec's apparent interest: whether, like me, she was hoping for more information on prognosis and treatment, or remembering what Kendrick had said, that palliative doctors were the pain specialists.

Sanjay pulled one of the green visitors' chairs as close to Cec's bed as he could and perched on the armrest. He was so tall that he still peered down at her but I appreciated his effort to get to her eye level.

"Dr. Kendrick reviewed the lab results with you?"

Cec nodded.

"The pathology report confirmed squamous cell carcinoma."

Uh-oh, I thought, I hope he's not just going to tell us what we already know.

"The cancer has metastasized." He paused.

What was he waiting for? We knew that the cancer had spread.

"And the appointment?" Cec said.

"Appointment?"

"With the oncologist."

"Oh. Yes."

"When is it?"

"Your appointment has been scheduled for March 10." This was the fourth.

"It can't be sooner?" I asked. Sanjay's head swiveled in my direction. "That's a long time to wait."

"I can check—"

"Or maybe you can tell us," Cec took a deep breath, "what happens now."

"The oncologist will be better able to answer your questions, about treatment options in particular."

"What's the prognosis? For this kind of cancer?" I asked. That was what Cec wanted to know.

"You'll be seeing Dr. Lillian Denton. She'll be able to give you a much better answer than I can."

"But Cec's appointment is a week away."

"That's the soonest—"

"Sooner," Cec said and closed her eyes. "We need to know."

"I'll see what I can do." Sanjay flipped through the papers in his hand. Something about the way he kept his head down told me that he wouldn't try to get her appointment moved up. And he still hadn't answered my question.

I tried a different approach. "Dr. Sanjay, it would help us both if we had an idea of what to expect, how this kind of cancer, squa—"

"Squamous cell carcinoma."

"Yes, how it normally progresses."

All I wanted was a simple prognosis!

"Well, uh, the cancer is aggressive."

"What does that mean?"

"It means the cancer has spread, in Cecile's case to her uterus. There's no evidence of cancer in her liver, or pancreas. This is a cancer that creates excess fluid. The fluid is putting pressure on her intestines. There are tumours around the bowels. We see some evidence of fluid collecting around the lungs."

"The flip side is the coin," Cec said, her tone firm. "You can't expect me to undo that!" She glared at Sanjay as she said this, her cheeks flushed.

"Does this happen frequently?" Sanjay looked at me and then at the IV monitor.

"Only on the dime," Cec said.

"We may need to change her to Hydromorph."

"Not without retribution!" Cec's eyes were fierce.

Sanjay hesitated. "Cecile, do you know where you are?"

"Of course."

"And what is your name?"

"Too simple," Cec said.

"My name is Dr. Sanjay."

"You just checked in."

"I'm checking in with you, to see how you are."

"Dull butter," or at least that's what it sounded like, then her eyes closed and her head fell back against the pillow.

"Cecile?" Sanjay touched her arm. Her eyes opened. "Would you like me to lower your morphine?"

She shook her head, no.

"If we bring your morphine dose down to five milligrams, it might help stop the hallucinations."

Cecile nodded and said what sounded like, "Surely."

Sanjay stood up, punched some buttons on the IV machine. "I'll put a note on her chart," he said.

After he left I stayed sitting beside her bed. I wanted to be there when she came back.

Cec opened her eyes, "Where'd he go?

"Sanjay? He left."

"He's a palliative doctor."

"Yes, he is."

"He gets the terminal cases."

"He does."

"Like me."

"Yes." I was relieved that she had put it together. The realization didn't seem to bother her.

"Have you called Doreen?" Cec asked.

"I have. She said to let you know that everyone is doing fine."

"She's keeping an eye on Ruby?"

"She is. But I should go out there."

"Not right now."

At some point I would have to leave her for a few hours to go out to the farm, even though she wouldn't want me to, and despite my own restless anxiety. I couldn't shake the feeling that life was coming unhinged, that reality was no longer completely reliable.

There was a part of me that knew my fears were on the edge of tipping over into the irrational. Paranoia. But I also knew that there existed a real possibility that a gate could be left open, or the dogs might wander. One of the cows might need help delivering her calf.

I'd asked Doreen to make sure that Ruby was contained in the small corral away from the other cows. I didn't want her having her baby out on the pasture. Annie had her first calf beside the creek.

When Annie didn't come up for her feed that evening, Cec did a scan of the pasture and spotted her on the far side of the creek.

We drove the half-ton down the slope of the gully on a rutted trail cut into the side of the hill. The creek was still partly frozen and we didn't want to chance getting stuck, so we parked the truck and walked across the lowest section of frozen creek bed, stepping from rock to rock, then across the wizened stubble to where Annie stood over her shivering newborn calf.

"Hey, good work ol' girl," Cec grinned. Annie stuck her big, wet nose into Cec's face. "It's all right, we're not going to hurt her. You need to let us help you. Not safe for you two out here."

Cec shooed Annie back so that I could pick up the calf—fifty pounds of wet, slippery hide over knobby knees and pointy hips. Cec ran interference, waving her arms to keep Annie from charging me, while I carried the calf with labouring, lumbering steps.

I made it across the creek without slipping on the ice or falling through (a minor miracle) and managed to heave the calf, now bawling, into the back of the truck. Then I crawled in after her and pushed the calf toward the truck cab where it would be easier for me to hang onto the truck and to her. Cec drove up the steep, bumpy incline as slowly as she could while still keeping up enough momentum to get up the last steep bit. Annie trotted along behind, tossing her head and bawling at us.

When we finally got Annie and her calf into the small corral and had shooed the other cows out, Annie seemed to forget that the calf was hers. She kicked at it when it tried to find a teat. It was such a wee bundle, wobbly and wet. A little heifer.

"Her name is River," Cec said.

"River?"

"She was born beside the creek but Creek isn't much of a name."

Cec found an old halter and we got it onto Annie, bribed her with oats, tied her to a post. The calf was skittish. We tried to nudge her toward her mama. Whenever the calf got close enough to lick Annie's teat, Annie would move her rump sideways or give a small kick. All the while she managed to keep her nose in the oats.

Cec looped a rope around one of Annie's back legs and lifted it a bit off the ground, enough that she was off balance and couldn't kick.

River found a teat and sucked, tongue flopping from side to side until she got it figured out. Then she gave Annie's udder a little head-butt. Annie stood still, her head turned so she could watch and complain. Her tone wasn't particularly motherly.

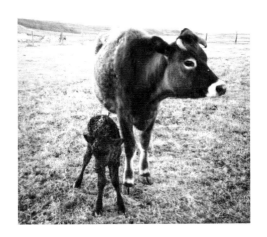

"Wish I'd paid closer attention."

Saturday, March 5

Each step down that long hallway was preparation—for whatever I'd find behind her door. Sometimes an empty bed when they'd taken her for tests. Sometimes a visitor and Cec at her charming morphined best. She heard every sound and knew when I came in, even when her eyes were closed.

This morning she was in bed. She turned to me without lifting her head from the pillow. She'd been waiting.

"I had a new nurse last night."

"Any good?"

"Allie. Gruff but sweet. She means well."

Maybe it was the sunlight pouring in through the window, or the way Cec's hair was a tousle of bed-head, but at that moment I saw Cec standing in front of the kitchen sink. She was wearing her plaid flannel shirt of deep blue and red, well worn, with a tear along one shoulder. When she turned I could see that the front was buttoned up lopsided. I couldn't help but grin.

"What are you laughing at?"

"You always button your shirts wrong."

Her designer-label suit jackets and silk shirts she would button up exactly right but her flannel chore shirts she often managed to button crooked. She'd lean against a counter or chair while I unbuttoned her shirt, and then re-buttoned it. When I was finished, she'd say, "Sanks, eh."

Cec's jaw clenched.

"Need more?"

A barely perceptible nod.

"I'll find her. Allie?"

"No. Day shift."

"Who is it?"

"Leave 'er."

Cec had done the math. She knew that she was just one more on a long list of cranky and bedridden.

"But you're in…"

"Don't want 'em mad at me."

When, in Cec's whole stubborn life, had she ever cared whether someone got mad at her? Even when she was a kid.

She said that she was nine, maybe ten, when her father started losing his vision. Macular degeneration. By the time Cec was twelve, or thirteen, he couldn't drive anymore and had enlisted Cec as his chauffeur. She was sturdy and willing. Her feet reached the pedals but she had to stand on the brake to come to a full stop.

He'd shown her how to clutch and shift, ease down on the brake. He always knew exactly where they were and would bark at her: "Slow down! Turn here!" He was a surly passenger and a sharp critic, unhappy at having to depend on a child.

Their errands frequently terminated at the Cecil Hotel in the rundown east end of Calgary's downtown. Cec would park behind the bar and wait in the truck while Jim sauntered in to "have a few with the boys." He was charming in a back-slapping, gruff sort of way and only got mean when he was drunk. Sometimes he didn't emerge from the Cecil until two or three in the morning. Cec would be fast asleep on the front seat, jerked awake by his pounding on the window.

One day when he'd been especially cranky about her driving she barked back, "Stop bossing me!"

He kept on.

She turned onto a side street and pulled over. "You want

to drive? I'll walk home. Leave you here."

He stopped then and sat staring out the window. She waited, to be sure.

And she still knew how to get what she wanted, even in her weakened state, from a hospital bed.

She could tell, for example, that I still wanted to go find her nurse, and she was keeping an eye on me.

"You need to call Doreen," she said, pointing for additional emphasis. She sounded lucid.

"I already did."

"Ask her if they can take the cows to auction."

"You want to sell the cows?" I was surprised, and felt an instant relief, followed immediately by hesitation. *Was she sure?* She had been adamant—"No! I'm not having this conversation!"—just a few weeks ago when I'd suggested we sell some of the animals.

"It's time."

It is? How do you know that? But I didn't ask. I just said, "Which ones?"

"All of them."

I couldn't have articulated it in that moment—I didn't consciously think the thought—but looking back I think I knew, in the way the body knows, without words, that she wasn't coming home to the farm again. And I knew that she knew.

"You can ask Doreen yourself," I said. "They're coming into Calgary today. She said they'd stop by."

A nurse I didn't recognize entered the room carrying a small paper cup filled with a yellow fluid. She was taller than average, and slender, with light-brown hair tied back into a ponytail.

"This stuff doesn't taste great, but it should help." Her voice was pleasant, soothing.

"Help what?"

"Get you moving."

"It all comes back up."

"Hopefully you can keep this down. We can try the other end too, if we need to. How's your pain?"

"About four. And I forgot your name."

"Kara."

"And you are…" Kara turned to me, "her sister?"

"I'm her partner." I had thought that this tidbit of information would have circulated among the nurses like it had among our country neighbours.

None of our neighbours had ever asked. Cec preferred to pretend that no one knew. I knew they did.

This was confirmed one evening when Hank and Doreen introduced us to friends of theirs while we were having dinner at the Country Cousins.

The woman said, "You live at the old Prohl place?"

We nodded.

The man squinted. "Oh, so you're the girls."

The yellow stuff didn't stay down, and I was ready with the basin.

Kara reappeared as I was handing Cec a glass of water to rinse her mouth.

"Here, I'll take that."

I gave her the basin and she disappeared through the bathroom door. A few minutes later she was back. "We'll try again."

"What's the point?"

"We need to keep trying. You're not going to feel better until you're moving again."

"It's been two days," I said.

"Hurts when I throw up." Cec was holding her stomach with both hands.

Kara put her stethoscope to Cec's belly.

"Trying to find a heartbeat?" Cec grimaced.

"Listening for a gurgle. Any sound is good—a fart, or a belch."

"I never fart," Cec said.

"Everyone farts."

"I don't."

I was tempted to tell Kara that it was true. I'd never heard Cec fart. She didn't sweat either, even after a day in the sun pulling weeds and hauling wheelbarrows full of dirt to build up the beds. The chestnut brown of her skin would deepen but no beads of sweat, no glowing forehead. When I wrapped my arms around her at the end of the day her skin was dry. This seemed to be a point of pride for her. I'd often wondered how her body regulated temperature, where her fluids went. They had to go somewhere.

Kara left to change a dressing, or empty a bedpan, or give a needle. I couldn't imagine coming in to work every day to deal with the blood, urine, pus-filled bandages, diarrhea, vomit ("emesis" they called it). There must be a desensitization process they put nurses through. Like those Halloween parties where someone blindfolds you and makes you stick your hands in bowls of Alpha-Getti or olives and tells you they are calf intestines or donkey testicles.

A small plastic cup of the yellow liquid that was supposed to get Cec moving was still sitting on her bedside table when my cell vibrated in my pocket. Cec hadn't thrown up for an hour. I stepped out of the room to answer. Mom and Dad were on their way up. They'd brought Noddy and wanted me to meet them at the elevators.

I'd asked Lorraine the day before whether I could bring Noddy in. She'd said that she couldn't give me permission but she would be willing to look the other way. To be on the safe side I should clear it with the head nurse. I had.

My mother was carrying Noddy in a tote bag over her shoulder. His head peeked out, ears perked. He craned his neck toward everyone he passed in case they wanted to pat him.

"Should I put his head in and zip him up?" Mom asked as we neared the doors to the ward.

"I don't think you need to. They know he's coming. But Cec doesn't."

I nudged Mom into the room first. I wanted her to have the pleasure of seeing Cec's expression when she saw Nod.

"Hey, my boy!"

He clambered out of the carrier.

"How are you, monkey?"

Noddy's tongue flapped in the direction of Cec's face. He was never very serious about landing a kiss.

Mom and Dad settled into the chairs at the foot of Cec's bed. Nod pranced down to the foot of the bed to give everyone a chance to pat his head.

"He believes in equal opportunity," Cec said. "Come here, fella."

"Lie down, Nod," I said.

"He's fine, Lyn."

Noddy sat on Cec's lap and thumped his head against her chest. Good therapy, I thought, to get a doggie hug.

"Lie down, buddy." I wanted him to curl up on her lap.

"He's okay." Cec was rubbing his head, her eyes closed. Her hand stopped moving. Her breathing paused.

"Lie down," I whispered to Nod, and he lifted his head in my direction. "No. Lie down." He waited to make sure I really meant it, then curled up on Cec's lap.

"He understands, doesn't he?" Mom said. "Sometimes I think he actually knows what we're saying to him."

"It's pretty amazing how such a small animal can communicate," Dad said, grinning. "He follows me around until I take him for a walk."

At the word "walk" Noddy lifted his head.

"No," I said, "you lie down." He lowered his head again.

Cec's breathing returned to normal, her hand continued

rubbing Nod's tummy. Footsteps and a quiet knock at Cec's hospital room door: Hank and Doreen.

"Is she sleeping?" Doreen's raspy whisper.

"I don't think so."

"Maybe we should come back another time."

"And miss the party?" Cec opened her eyes and waved them into the room.

"Doreen, this is my mom, Mary, and my dad, Richard. And this is Hank." Hank smiled shyly. He was tall with a high, wide forehead and ruddy complexion, large work-worn hands.

Doreen handed Cec an envelope. "How are you?"

"I've had better days." Cec opened the card, read it, and laid it on her lap. "Thank you."

I would rescue the card from Cec, eventually, and stand it up on the windowsill with the other cards. Whenever Cec got out of bed or sat with her legs hanging over the bed on the side nearest the window, she'd knock the row of cards over. If she managed to flick the first one, the rest would fall like dominoes. The next time I was opening or closing the shutters, I'd stand the cards back up again.

Doreen was beside Cec's bed, Noddy nudging Doreen's hand with his head.

"You're the Loewens?" my dad asked. I'd told Mom and Dad about Hank and Doreen helping us with chores, but they'd never met. "Do you have relatives in Manitoba?" My father couldn't help himself. Hank nodded. "Loewen" is a distinctly Mennonite last name.

"Probably there are," Hank said, "but no *Frintschoft*" (the Low German word for relative). "My mother was a Toews," Hank said, "and Doreen is from PEI. She's Scottish."

"Like me," Cec piped up.

"You doing all right in here?" Doreen patted Cec's blanketed foot.

"For an old girl."

"Will they let you go home?"

"I don't know. I'd like to…"

While Doreen talked to Cec, I kept hearing Kendrick's voice: *Palliative. Stage four. Squamous cell carcinoma.* I sat silently, with a gnawing dread.

"Maybe we should go," Mom said. "I'm not sure how long the nurses will let Noddy stay."

"As long as he wants." Cec pulled Noddy closer.

"We don't want to tire you out," Doreen said.

"Stay!" Cec said, in as firm a voice as she could manage. "The cows—" Cec nudged me.

"Oh yeah. Doreen. We're wondering whether you could take the cows to auction."

"Which ones?" She was instantly all business.

"All of them."

"Even the little bull?"

Cec's eyes were closed but she was nodding. Sham was our little Dexter bull. He had a knack for sidestepping the loading chute.

"The auction is on Tuesday," Hank said. "We'd have to take them on Monday."

I suddenly felt like crying. I'd said to Cec, several times over the last months, that I thought we should sell some animals. Chores took a couple of hours every day and feed was expensive. Cec had stormed off, unwilling to entertain the idea of selling even a single goat, and now she was telling Doreen to sell the cows, all of them.

Cec's eyes rolled up into the back of her head. Her breathing stopped.

"She comes back," I said. "It just takes a while. If I can count to ten, I'm supposed to go get the—"

Cec's eyes rolled forward. She took a breath. "You'll be able to load him," she said. "He's a good boy."

Later that evening, when Cec was sleeping and the ward was quiet, I walked out into the main hallway and dialed Doreen's cellphone.

When I heard her voice, my throat tightened.

"She's pretty bad, eh."

"Yeah, she is."

"Don't worry about the cows. We'll take them on Monday."

My throat tightened again. The next time I'd drive onto the yard, the corrals would be empty.

"The dogs, Doreen, I want to put them in the kennel."

"I don't think they'll wander."

I wasn't so sure. I hadn't been home for almost a week. They might get restless and I knew the neighbours wouldn't tolerate roving dogs, especially at calving time. A strange dog wandering through a pasture or farmyard was at risk of being shot on sight, no questions asked.

"I just don't know how much longer…" Another catch in my throat. "If I call the kennel, would you take them?"

"I don't know about having them in the half-ton. Griff's pretty big."

"Take our van. The keys are in it. Griff will hop in no problem. Charlie doesn't like cars much. You might have to lift her."

I'm watching golf as I write this. One year later. Tiger is leading. That would have made Cec happy. The muted drone of golf commentary is comforting. I'm sitting at the dining room table reading through Cec's medical records: a copy from her family doctor, her file from the Didsbury doctor, a thick folder from the hospital. I've three-hole-punched the pages, put them in a burgundy binder, labeled the spine:

MEDICAL RECORDS – CECILE KAYSOE – 2005

Some of the handwriting is almost illegible but I can follow the notes from the night Cec was admitted. The hospital record charts her pain, her level of coherency, absence of bowel movements, who was visiting, her medications.

20:00 – Patient still complaining of escalating pain. 5 mg morphine given. Continue to assess pain and offer morphine as required. Patient refuses to try Ibuprofen. States, "It doesn't do anything."

I flip to the page that lists which nurse administered the medications on which day. These notes were written by Allie. She had that instinct some nurses have, about touch and timing. What had put me at ease even more was that I could tell right away that Allie liked Cec.

23:30 – Patient pain remains uncontrolled. Morphine not

effective. Resident paged. Lactulose 15 ml given for bloating. Continue to monitor.

Where was I? Probably asleep at Mom and Dad's.

00:10 – Hydromorph 2 mg tab given for pain. Pain remains uncontrolled ~ 7/10. Patient restless, unable to settle. States Hydromorph "makes me feel dopey but doesn't take pain away." Patient refuses hot/cold packs and Ibuprofen.

None of the doctors had said anything about how mad the cells of the body can get when they are surgically invaded. Or how, in the case of malignancy, an invasion can rile up cancer cells. No one said anything about how anesthetic makes the bowels sluggish or that obstructions are not uncommon.

Did they know their surgical exploration could ratchet up her pain? Or how dire the ultimate consequence might be?

Sunday, March 6

"Hand me that notebook, would you?" Cec pointed at her bedside table. "I made you a list. What you need to get."

Small transistor radio (so she could listen to Stuart McLean)

Depends diapers

Bottled water—flat of Co-op Gold

Newspaper

I had picked up a paper on my way in that morning, and I'd stopped at the bank. The night before Cec had given me her debit card, her password, and a list of bills to pay. She wasn't sure of the amounts owing, told me to put $500 on each so we'd be covered.

"You should be able to get all of this at London Drugs," Cec said. "There's one on 32nd Avenue. Use my debit card."

"I can pay."

"We may as well spend the money in my account," she said, "seeing as I have some. Hand me my purse."

I got her purse out of the small locker in the corner of her room. She pulled out her debit card and her cheque book.

"What are you doing?"

"Making sure you have cash."

She handed me two cheques for $3000 each. "There's enough in my chequing to cover those. Put them in your wallet. Just in case."

"One paycheque away," Cec would say, usually on the heels of a conversation about the shingles that had blown off the barn roof or the call she'd made to Virgil to bring another load of bales.

"If you lose your job, or I do," she'd say, "or one of us gets sick, that's it, we'll be out on the street pushing a grocery cart. We're two educated, successful career women, but we're just like everyone else, leveraged to the hilt."

I was never sure whether she actually meant what she was saying. She seemed so relaxed about it, half joking. I had a vague idea about how much she earned—upwards of $100,000 plus bonuses and benefits. Hers was a managerial position so she wasn't paid commission even though she personally managed the large projects. But her bonuses were sizeable, at least that's the impression she gave off. I didn't look at her pay stubs, never opened her mail, even when the registered letters from the Canada Revenue Agency, the tax collectors, started to arrive.

It was my job, on Saturdays, to take the old half-ton into town for the mail, drop garbage at the dump, and in the summertime get gas in the red jerry cans for the lawn mower and garden tractor. I didn't think much about the first registered letter—handed it to Cec with the other envelopes. When the second one arrived, a couple weeks later, I said to her, "What is this? I had to sign for it."

She waved me off, "It's nothing."

"Registered mail from the tax department isn't nothing." I didn't usually comment on, or ask about, money, or mail, or credit cards or bank accounts. We had separate accounts and she hated being questioned—said it made her feel as though I didn't trust her—but the words just came out.

Surprisingly, she answered: "They screwed up at work. We were audited and the CRA said our HR department made a mistake, something about the way they were allocating expenses. It's not my problem. They have to fix it."

The registered letters kept coming. I continued to sign for them. A couple of months later, I asked her again about the letters.

"It's not my problem." She waved me off.

Her answer didn't sit right, but I didn't challenge her. She was good with numbers, paid bills on time, found her way through complicated project calculations. And she was stubborn. If she didn't think she should have to pay, she would dig in her heels. Maybe the results of the audit were being reviewed, or contested. She would give me sufficient warning if it was time to search out a suitable shopping cart.

We were downtown one afternoon when she said, "This would be a good spot."

"For what?"

"That corner," she said, pointing. "We'd have Noddy with us. People like little dogs. We wouldn't go hungry."

I could imagine it. Cec wouldn't beg. She'd smile and make some offhand comment. She wouldn't seem particularly destitute or deprived, just worn around the edges. She'd engage the ones who smiled. They'd find themselves telling her about their dog or the time they'd taken home a stray.

"Your job would be bottle collection," she said.

"Yes, I'm good at that," I said, still not sure how seriously to take her. I was the one who insisted we collect our empties. Cec would throw them out.

"But they're worth money," I'd say, indignant, as I pulled the empties out of the garbage.

Cec thought it funny in a charming sort of way, my determination to take our bottles back, and my satisfaction with the resulting fistful of change.

"It's not as though we're on the verge of homelessness." I knew better than to put it to her as a question. Cec had taught me this: Don't ask a question. Make a statement. That's what men do. They make statements, even when they know that what they're saying is bullshit. Men test the waters, watch for reactions. Women ask questions, very sincere questions, the kind that telegraph motivations and uncertainties.

"Not time to find a shopping cart yet," Cec said, "but the farm is an expensive hobby. There are days when I think it would be easier to be a bag lady."

I was surprised to hear this, coming from her. She was adamant that she'd never move off the farm. "You seem to enjoy the idea," I said, "of living on the street."

"It would be a kind of freedom."

"Most people think of pushing a grocery cart as failure."

She shrugged. "Money is just money. I've lived with a lot of money and I've lived with a little. Truth is, there's not much difference."

Cec's gynecologist came by at noon. I'd gone down to the cafeteria to get a sandwich and was on my way back when I saw a man in scrubs with a wrinkly green O.R. cap on his head. He backed out of Cec's room and closed the door behind him. I didn't know that he was Cec's gynecologist, and kicked myself later that I hadn't made it back a few minutes sooner. I couldn't count on Cec to give me a reliable report.

What I really wanted to know was why he had never—in all his consultations with Cecile, and especially as her pain got worse—tested her for cancer. Or maybe he had and Cec hadn't told me? That was a possibility. Not easy to ask her now; she was so often in a mental fog and I didn't want to upset her fragile equilibrium with questions that might sound like accusation.

I imagined training my eyes on her gynecologist, calm and steady, as I asked him why no one had explained to Cecile, or to me, that if the mass on her ovary was cancerous and especially if the cancer had spread, that any kind of invasive procedure might make it worse? It seemed to me that that was exactly what had happened; her tumours had started producing fluid at an accelerated rate after the surgery.

Was he a gyne-oncologist? No? Then why hadn't he referred her to one?

I'd rehearsed my questions, imagined my conversation with him, but I hadn't actually expected him to show up. A part of me was glad that we'd passed each other silently in the hallway. I was too tired for confrontation. I wouldn't have been able to keep my voice steady.

Cec had another round of throwing up. She was white and exhausted. I waited until it looked as though she had fallen asleep, or at least her version of sleep, and tiptoed out of her room. I needed to get out. Those pale-blue walls were making me feel as though we were living in a fish bowl.

I slumped into an empty wheelchair outside her door. The hum of the internal air circulation system of the hospital worked on me like a cocoon. I didn't notice Mom until she sat down beside me.

"How is she?" Mom was whispering.

"Sleeping, I think."

"Would this be a good day for me to apologize?"

"Anytime her eyes are open, and she doesn't seem to be in too much pain, will be as good a time as any."

I heard what sounded like the movement of blankets from behind Cec's half-closed door. "Lyn?"

I went back into her room.

"Hey, you're awake," I said, with more energy than I felt.

"Are you feeling any better?" My mother, the eternal optimist, was right behind me.

"I don't know," Cec said. "On a scale of one to ten what is 'better'?" She pointed at her IV machine. "How much am I getting? Can you find Kara?"

As I left the room, I heard Mom say, "Cecile, I know this probably isn't the best time…"

No, Mom, it's probably not, I thought to myself, but you might as well say what you have to say.

Later Cec said, "Did she tell you that she was going to…" then her jaw clenched.

"Apologize? Yes. What did she say?"

"Made a pretty heavy go of it, like it was a school project."

"She said she needed to."

"Not for my sake."

"I told her you were past that."

"Was she afraid she'd have a blemish on her record?"

"I think she's truly sorry."

A little while later, as I sat staring out the window at a cloudy sky, Cec said, "Nothing like a weepy apology to make you feel like you really are on your last legs."

I waited. I could sense her mind churning.

"When my mother…" Cec held her stomach, talking as she grimaced, "…was ill, I thought she was my lesson in aging." She sucked in a deep breath, held it, exhaled with a shudder. "I didn't realize she was…" Her mouth fell open, eyes rolled up. I waited. Her eyes came forward again, "… my apprenticeship in dying." She gave a wry smile. "Wish I'd paid closer attention."

It's the middle of the afternoon and I've come into Calgary to do a few errands. I should be at home mowing the lawn but I don't have the energy. The farmyard seems large and empty now that the llamas and horses are gone. I wonder how long I will be able to stand living out there by myself.

Mom has been cleaning cupboards but she needs to take a break, she says. She's making herself some decaf coffee. I make myself a cup of tea and settle into a patio chair on Mom and Dad's newly expanded deck.

Mom sets a plate of her homemade chocolate-and-peanut-butter fibre squares beside me. Dark chocolate contains antioxidants, fibre an important part of any breakfast, protein in the peanut butter. Entirely justifiable.

I hold a chocolate square between my finger and thumb. The chocolate starts to melt.

Mom pushes the patio table and the chocolate squares closer to me and straightens the chairs. She goes back inside for a damp cloth and wipes down the table. "So hard to keep these clean."

Eventually she sits down and takes a chocolate for herself.

"I had a dream last night," she says, "and I woke up thinking about you."

"Oh?"

"You weren't in it but I wanted to tell you." She takes a small bite of her chocolate and I wait for her to finish chewing. "I dreamt that I was getting married to a woman."

"A woman? Really?!" I knew that my mother didn't view same-sex relationships as an aberration anymore, but I still

wouldn't ever have imagined having this conversation. She doesn't seem upset, or even embarrassed.

"Do you know Rosalyn?"

"No, I don't think so."

"She's just been through a terrible divorce from a very abusive man. She's the one I was getting married to."

"And you were…?" I was still surprised that Mom seemed so completely okay with this.

"I was in a car and I was trying to find my parents' house because all my clothes were there, and my wedding dress. Rosalyn was already at the church. She was so excited about getting married. I was worried that the church wouldn't allow the wedding to go ahead."

"And did they?"

"I don't know. I couldn't find my parents' house. I didn't have any clothes on and I didn't have my wedding dress. I went back to the church. I was naked but I didn't care."

"You didn't?" In real life she certainly would have.

"I really didn't."

"Did you get married naked?"

"When I walked into the church it was full of women. They were there to help us get ready. And one of them, I don't remember who, said to me, 'You don't have any clothes on but you look quite comfortable.' And it was true."

I was glad to see Allie's dependable round face. She checked Cec's vitals and asked about her pain.

Cec said her pain was a six. That made me sit up. Cec almost never admitted to anything above a four.

"We could boost your morphine to ten for a while—"

"No." Cec was on the verge of tears. "I just want to stop throwing up."

"Mmmm." Allie pursed her lips. "I have an idea. Be back in a minute."

When Allie came back, about ten minutes later, Melinda the head nurse, short and matronly, was with her.

"Allie says you're not keeping anything down."

Cec nodded.

"I think we should pump her stomach," Allie said in her no-nonsense way.

"Pump her stomach?"

"If we pump your stomach you won't have anything left to throw up." Allie waited for a response. Cec looked at me.

"It's up to you," I said.

"We'd insert a tube into your nose and down," Allie pointed toward her nose, then curled her finger downwards. "We'd hook you up to a pump and suck out whatever you have left in there."

"Will it hurt?" Cec asked.

"You'll barely feel anything."

"How long will it take?"

"A few hours. The suction pressure will be light."

"If I do this," Cec turned to me, "I'd want you to stay."

"Of course."

"For the night."

"You could sleep in her bed," Allie said to me. Then to Cec, "It would work best if you were in a recliner. That way we could move you closer to the wall. We'll need to attach the tube to that container." She pointed at a clear plastic container that was mounted to the wall.

"I would assist," the head nurse said.

I wanted to ask how they could be sure they wouldn't push the tube into Cec's lungs but I kept my mouth shut. They'd done this before. There was a way, I was sure. I knew that Doreen had put tubes down into the stomachs of newborn calves to force feed them. If Doreen could do that, Allie could do this.

"If I'm going to stay, I should call Mom," I said to Cec. I had no desire to watch while they put the tube in.

"Go ahead," Allie said. "This won't take long."

I was on my way back to Cec's room when I saw him standing at the nurses' station, his back to me. He seemed stocky but then he straightened. He was tall, slender, his white lab coat swaying like a choir gown. He had a blue tensor bandage around one wrist and was carrying a white plastic case with a LAB SERVICES label on the side. A perfect cover, I thought. He could be carrying a syringe and vials of strychnine. No, that was for gophers. He looked up. *Did he see the question in my eyes?* I hadn't figured out Plan B. Something not too messy. *Was it possible to end a human life without it getting messy?*

I looked away, my cheeks hot. *Could he read the guilt in my eyes?*

A nine-inch length of tubing with a knob on the end was hanging out of one of Cec's nostrils.

Allie rolled a pink vinyl recliner from the hallway into the room. We pushed Cec's bed against the window so the recliner could be positioned as close as possible to the container on the wall. Allie covered the recliner with a sheet, then a blanket. Together we helped Cec from the bed to the chair. It was surprisingly easy to move Cec with Allie helping even though Cec barely moved her feet.

Allie attached the tube dangling out of Cec's nose to a longer tube that was attached to the clear container. She turned a dial. The pump started up, a low hum, like the churn of the pump in our wellhouse.

A thin stream of orangey-brown liquid began moving along the tube.

"What is that?" I ask Allie.

"That's what was in her stomach."

I hadn't expected her stomach contents to look so orange. Cec lifted the tubing and watched the liquid swirl along.

"Does it hurt?" I asked her.

She shook her head.

I changed into a T-shirt and pajama bottoms and crawled on top of the blankets on Cec's hospital bed. The lights in the room were out except for the greenish light from the IV monitor and a wash of grey light seeping in from the hallway. The IV machine beeped rhythmically. Cec was tipped back in the recliner, her eyes closed, her breathing shallow. The stomach pump pumped, a low groan. I lay on my side, facing her. She looked so fragile. I was afraid that if I closed my eyes she might dissolve. But I couldn't stare at her every minute. I let my eyes fall shut and lay still.

Allie checked in on us at regular intervals. If it looked as though we were both sleeping, she'd check the fluid in the container and Cec's IV and leave again. I lay absolutely still and completely aware, like a German shepherd guard dog. When she opened her eyes, Cec would reach for my hand. Her touch was cool, her fingers weightless. I held her hand and closed my eyes, my ears tuned to the rise and fall of her breaths.

In my heavy-headed half-dream lethargy, I thought I saw smoke curling out of Cec's mouth. I opened my eyes. Her head was tipped back, mouth open. No smoke.

I closed my eyes again, let my mind sink into the mud of half-sleep. In my semi-conscious dream, Cec sat up in her recliner and lit a cigarette. She was talking to someone. I couldn't see who it was but I knew that it was Christian, the guy whose engagement proposal she hadn't accepted. He was behind the curtain. I couldn't hear what Cec was saying to him and when he spoke all I heard was a rumble of unintelligible syllables. I wanted to ask him whether he had brought her box from Denmark. Cec told me once that she had written a novel and that her manuscript was in one of the boxes she had stored at Christian's. I tried to say *Did you bring the box?* but my mouth wouldn't form the words.

Monday, March 7

By morning about an inch of orangey-brown liquid had gathered in the container. Cec said she needed to go to the washroom. I put on my glasses, a sweater, and slippers and went to find Allie. I'd thought about pushing the CALL button, but Cec didn't like to ring for the nurses. She preferred to dispatch her messenger.

Allie turned off the pump and unhooked Cec, left the tube dangling from her nose. I unplugged the IV machine and pulled her recliner upright as smoothly as I could. I could tell that Allie had hoped for better output from Cec's stomach. She didn't say anything, but I saw the way she examined the contents of the container, with a furrowed brow and a slight frown.

The lab tech knocked timidly on the door, a slight girl in a too-large lab coat, sleeves rolled up. Her black, shiny hair was scooped into a straying pile at the back of her head and she carried a white plastic container filled with syringes and small vials of blood.

She nodded a quiet hello and made her way around to the far side of Cec's bed. Left arm. She should have stopped and asked (with the greeting I thought they'd all been trained to softly exhale), "Which arm?"

She would discover, when she pulled up the sleeve of Cec's gown, that the inner bend of her elbow and the soft patch of skin that ran to the inner wrist was red-pricked and blue-welted, one vein bulging, her skin a feverish pink.

I realized, watching the lab techs inspect Cec's welts, that I didn't turn away or close my eyes. When the nurses would change the dressing under Cec's arm, the oozing seepage from the blood-encrusted wound didn't make me queasy. It's the animals, I thought. The farm had toughened me. All those years of watching baby animals be born, putting salve on sores and cuts, tending calves with diahrrea, I'd gotten used to the sight of blood and bodily fluids.

The lab tech's brow furrowed as she wrapped a tourniquet just above the elbow of Cec's left arm. Cec clenched her jaw. The ones with the lightest touch often had the greatest trouble plunging the needle in with exact force.

The lab tech swabbed. Small fingers. Child hands. She looked eighteen or nineteen. She fit a needle onto the end of a small vial and pressed Cec's skin with her thumb. She pressed again, a little more firmly, and watched for the blue pop of a vein. She pressed one more time, needle tip pointed toward the ceiling. Cec tensed in anticipation.

When she pushed the needle into Cec's arm, Cec grimaced but made no sound.

"Oh!" the young girl said, with faint surprise. She withdrew the needle, swabbed a new location, and jabbed again.

"Aahh," from Cec. The lab tech was moving the needle tip in Cec's arm trying to nick a vein. Cec reached for me and I grabbed her hand. She squeezed *hard*.

The lab tech eventually managed to extract the required vials of blood. She closed her box and left Cec to press a small wad of cotton against another puffing welt. Cec examined the wound in her arm and rolled her eyes.

I was feeling a little queasy. The blood I could handle but not the butchering of the extraction. It was the same spinning sensation I'd had the day Cec decided it was time to trim Annie's horns.

Cec and I had said to each other in passing that Annie's horns needed trimming. They'd grown long and were curling round, would soon penetrate her skull. One hot July afternoon Cec announced it was time.

She shooed the other cows out of the corral and, with the help of a bucket of oats, I coaxed Annie up the shoot until she got to the headstall. Cec pulled the lever that moved the metal frames into position around Annie's neck, not too tight, to hold her head in place.

Cec brought out an array of saws from her collection, some too large, others too dull. The little blue hacksaw had the sharpest teeth and was the easiest to use, although it still felt rather precarious to be wielding such a sharp blade so close to a live, mooing head. Cec found an angle that would work for both her arms and the safety of Annie's head. I held Annie's halter to make sure her head stayed still. A little sweat and muscle and the top four inches of the first horn were severed.

"Your turn," Cec said.

We traded places. I eyeballed a place on the second horn that I thought would make it about even with the first, and started to saw, tentatively at first, but then picked up a bit of speed. The blade slid easily and Annie was still busy getting as many oats into her mouth as possible.

A spurt of blood.

I stopped. We looked at each other. My work gloves and the front of my coveralls were covered in blood.

"Guess you're a bit farther down than you should be."

"But I thought—"

Cec shook her head. "Nothing to do but keep going. It's already done. You're not hurting her."

I kept going. Blood spurted and gushed. Annie seemed unconcerned. When bloody spatter hit my face, I said to Cec, "I can't. You have to."

We took turns, each of us sawing until the blood on our clothes, and on the top of Annie's caramel-brown head, made our knees go weak. All through my last turn with the saw, I was crying. My limbs were rubber.

"Don't!" Cec said.

"I can't help it." I wiped tears from my face with the back of my bloody glove.

"You look like you just butchered something." She was laughing.

"Don't make me laugh, I have to finish."

When the horn was finally severed, I fell to the ground. My hands were shaking. I was breathing hard, and half-smiling at Cec through a blur of tears. "Shit! I can't believe it."

"You did great."

"I feel like I'm going to puke."

"We'd make lousy chainsaw murderers."

Sanjay arrived just after Cec's breakfast tray had been deposited on her bedside table. Jell-O, Boost, Cheerios. Cec turned up her nose.

Behind Sanjay, there was another doctor. He was young, and short, not more than 5'2." He walked with the stiff stride of a bodybuilder, obviously conscious of his muscles.

Sanjay nodded at Cec, and at me, "Good morning. This is Dr. Daniel Steader. He will be managing your care. This is Cecile. And this is Lyn, Cecile's partner."

Steader nodded. He stepped up to the side of Cec's bed. "I'll be taking over for Dr. Kendrick. Dr. Sanjay will continue to consult with regard to pain management. How are you feeling this morning?"

"Better. After the pump." Cec gestured toward the plastic container on the wall. Allie had cleaned it out and set it back in its place.

"How bad is your pain, on a scale of—"

Cec held up three fingers.

"Do you mind if I have a listen?" Steader put his stethoscope to his ears and pulled Cec's blanket away but didn't lift her nightie. He pressed the stethoscope to her belly on top of her hospital gown.

I sat in a chair at the foot of Cec's bed while he asked about her bowel movements, the frequency of her vomiting, the enemas, the pumping of her stomach.

I still wanted to know about prognosis. I hoped Cec would ask. She hadn't asked when Kendrick gave her the diagnosis and got irritated when I pushed for information.

Steader pulled Cec's blanket back up over her belly, "Has anyone spoken with you about levels of care?"

Cec shook her head.

"They are essentially three levels of intervention. In the case of a life-threatening event such as a heart attack, for instance, we need to know whether you want us to intervene, and to what extent."

"Like a DNR?" I asked.

"Level three is a DNR. There would be no life-saving measures."

"And Level two?"

"Level two involves non-invasive procedures, but not surgery, for example, or life support. Level one includes all possible restorative measures."

Steader looked at Cec, waiting for a response. I was waiting too. She looked back at us without expression.

Why was she not responding? Hadn't she been adamant that she wasn't planning to hang around? What about Plan B? Maybe it was the morphine.

"It's important that you make your wishes known to your family," Steader said when Cec remained silent, "or those who may have to make decisions regarding your care."

Cec didn't respond. Steader was about to speak again when Cec said, "You people don't understand." She tapped her head with her index finger. "I'm operating at about fifteen percent..." She closed her eyes. "Don't like not knowing."

"Okay," Steader said, "I'll leave the information with your friend, and you can let the nurse know when you've made a decision. There's a document you'll need to sign."

"I would also recommend," Sanjay stepped forward, "that we change you over to Fentanyl. Narcotics have a tendency to build up in the bloodstream. Eventually the side effects, such as the hallucinations, override the benefits."

Cec opened her eyes again. "Can't decide." She looked like she might cry.

"A change in meds may alleviate some of your discomfort." Sanjay turned to locate his clipboard.

"Not now," Cec said.

"Give it some thought."

They left. No one had said anything about prognosis.

"Why didn't you ask?" I said to Cec.

"About what?"

"Prognosis."

"Doesn't matter."

"It doesn't?" It did to me.

"I don't think they know."

"What don't they know?"

She leaned back against her pillow. "This isn't going to end well."

Cec was sucking a blue Popsicle when I went down to the cafeteria for breakfast. She might sip some Boost but she wouldn't touch the Jell-O or the Cheerios. I kept imagining bits of Cheerio getting sucked out of Cec's stomach through the tube that was still hanging out of her nose.

On my way back to the ward, I pulled my cellphone out of my pocket, my only connection to the outside world. I was shuffling along the wide outer hallway—"the racetrack" as Cec called it—that connected the four wards, one ward entrance at each corner of the rectangular hallway.

Most of the people that I passed were from the outside world. They were easily identifiable: untethered to IV poles, carrying flowers, walking with purpose. I didn't meet their eyes, looked out the grimey windows—*someone should clean them*—away from the peach-coloured walls, almost pink. The colour of the walls made me think of skin. My mind went from skin to intestines and from there to vomit and directly to Pepto-Bismol. Whenever I walked down the hall, I got that pepperminty taste of Pepto-Bismol in my mouth.

I flipped open my cellphone. There was a message waiting from Tom. How had I missed it?

He was sorry to hear about Cecile. He hoped I was doing okay. Could I please call him? Reliance Energy had some questions. He needed to know how long I'd be away.

I had just submitted a console bid for half a million dollars to Reliance. It was a good sign they had questions. But Tom didn't know the details.

I dialed Tom's number. I couldn't go into the office, not for more than an hour. I'd need half a day to deal with the Reliance bid. He wouldn't be happy about that. And I needed to ask for a leave of absence. It was pretty much impossible to predict his response. It would depend on his mood, his frame of mind in the moment.

If he didn't give me a leave, would I have to quit? Could he fire me? What would we live on if I wasn't working?

I thought about the envelopes from the CRA and wished I'd opened one. Just one. The CRA doesn't send multiple registered letters without a good reason. There was something she wasn't telling me. Until this moment, I had been fine not knowing.

Lora arrived after lunch. She had taken another day off work. Couldn't concentrate, she said, would rather sit with Cec.

"I have to go," I said, and didn't wait for a response. I walked past Lora and out the door before Lora had even said hello to Cec. I needed to find Marion. I often met her in the elevator or passed her in the hallway. She might be in the cafeteria. I walked quickly, almost running. She was at her office door, inserting the key.

"I need to talk to you." I was breathless.

"About what?"

Instant tears. *Shit!*

"Come in."

She led me through an office space with several desks behind partitions and into a room with a couch, two chairs, two coffee tables, a small table with a coffee maker and a tissue box. The minute I sat down on the couch my eyes filled with tears. Marion handed me a tissue.

"How are you holding up?"

"About like this, except I don't cry in her room. She hates it when I cry."

"Mmmm, and can you do that?"

"What? Not cry?"

She nodded.

"Sometimes I have to leave the room."

"It's natural."

"What is?"

"Your tears. It's called anticipatory grief."

Grief? I stared at the tissue in my hand. "But—she's still—" *Really? Was this grief?*

Marion handed me the tissue box and moved the garbage can closer. "It's okay to cry."

Fresh tears. My nose wouldn't stop running. I felt like a traitor, crying like this, and talking to Marion.

"The weekend was awful." I shuddered then inhaled a

deep breath. "She wouldn't stop throwing up so they put a tube down her nose and pumped her stomach."

I blew my nose again. Marion waited. The room was absolutely quiet—no footsteps, no voices, no IV machines beeping.

"The worst part is that no one will tell us anything."

"What do you mean?"

"The palliative doctor. Sanjay. You know him. You must. All the people you've seen die…" I took a deep breath.

She didn't say anything.

"I need you to talk to him. When we ask about prognosis all he will say is that we should talk to the oncologist. But the appointment isn't until Thursday! That's three days away. I need to know now." My face was hot. "I need you to tell him to talk to us."

"They haven't said anything about prognosis?"

"No. We've asked several times, but no one will say, straight out, how bad it is."

Marion was sitting across from me, several feet away but I had the sense that, if she could have reached, she would have taken hold of my hands. I was shivering, even though I wasn't cold. Fury had drained my strength.

"I'm not a medical doctor," she said slowly, choosing her words. "I haven't read Cecile's chart, but from what I've observed, from what I know of her situation, it looks to me as though she doesn't have much time left."

Marion saw the question in my eyes.

"I don't know," she said. "I can't say whether it's days or weeks, but it's not long." She paused to let her words sink in as I dried my eyes, then continued, "Does she have a will?"

"Yes."

"You know where it is?"

"I have it." The clinical calm of her voice was beginning to settle me.

"Have you talked with her about her wishes?"

"Mostly. But there are still some details…I need to ask."

Marion sat up. I half-expected her to get out a piece of paper and make a list. The heat had dissipated from my face. My eyes were sore and puffy, but my cheeks were dry.

"Get all the paperwork together," she said in a low voice, as though we were co-conspirators. "Do that as soon as you can. Do you have her papers here?"

"They're at the farm."

"Then go get them, as soon as you can, today or tomorrow. Don't put this off. Go through them with her. Make all the arrangements. Have you talked with a funeral home?"

"No." I swallowed. For a moment I couldn't breathe.

Her voice was gentle, "This isn't easy, I know."

"Feels wrong when she's still alive."

"It will be easier for you if you do it now. You won't be in a good frame of mind later." She paused again. "Take care of the arrangements, and then spend as much time as you can with her. Say what you need to say. Don't leave it. People think that there will be time, right at the end. They hold off, waiting for the right moment to say those precious final words, but that's not how it works. A dying person begins to separate."

"I think it's already happening."

"At the very end, the world of a dying person becomes very small. All they have energy for is what is absolutely necessary. Often they aren't able to carry on a conversation. Keep that in mind. You don't have much time. Be with her as much as you can."

I sat with my head bowed staring at the bunched-up tissues in my hands.

"Okay." I took a deep breath and stood up. She lifted the wastebasket and I dropped my used tissues in.

"You'll talk to Sanjay?" I asked.

"I'll see what I can do."

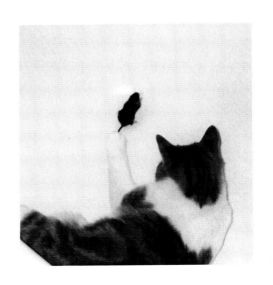

"Only Females"

Tuesday, March 8

I spent a second night lying perfectly still on Cec's bed. I must have slept. When I opened my eyes the window was filled with wispy clouds, a hazy light. Cec was in her recliner, tipped back as far as it would go, swaddled in blankets, her eyes open.

"I couldn't sleep," she said. "I wanted to be in my bed but you were there."

"You should have woken me."

"You were asleep."

"Next time wake me."

"Not if you're sleeping."

"Even if I'm sleeping!"

"Don't do this, Lyn!"

"Do what?"

No response. Her eyes closed again.

I shuffled into the cafeteria, eyes on the floor. I was wearing my pajama bottoms and the bulky red fleece that Cec hated. I had put on a baseball cap to hide my bed-head.

I sat staring at a paper bowl filled with hot, lumpy oatmeal. I added brown sugar and milk. I couldn't eat. The thought of chewing made me tired.

I left my uneaten bowl of oatmeal and headed back toward the elevator, measuring my progress with my peripheral vision. The stairs were to my left, the elevators straight ahead. The

UP button had already been pushed. I heard fragments of conversation, voices speaking in confidential tones. Often there was a crush of bodies that would shove toward the elevator door when it *pinged* and slid open. If a shoulder bumped against my shoulder, I wouldn't look up. I didn't say sorry. If anyone looked at me, they saw a bowed head, shuffling steps.

The elevator door opened. I stepped in. No jostling of shoulders or baby carriages today. No sharp scent of the cold spring air that visitors bring in with them. But I was not alone. A woman stood to one side, close to the buttons. I knew she was a woman by the pointed toes of her black winter boots and the black wool pants that hung, perfectly hemmed, just at the top of her three-inch heels.

My eyes travelled to her waist. She was average height, and slight, wearing a red-felt winter coat. I glanced up at her face. I couldn't help myself, a quick peek at the cut of her hair, the shade of her lipstick. I found myself looking into dark-brown eyes. She didn't blink.

My vision went blurry. I looked back down at my feet.

She said, "Do you need a hug?"

A hug? She didn't say, *Are you okay?* the fallback question of those caught off guard by tears. This was the main reason I kept my eyes averted: so no one would feel obliged to ask.

The carefully tailored woman was waiting for me to answer. I nodded.

She reached up. I bent down. She wrapped her arms around me and hugged me tight. There was a moment of solace in the strength of her embrace.

The elevator door opened. She touched my arm with her gloved hand then stepped out. One backward glance and she was gone.

I took a deep breath. I had not dissolved or blubbered. In fact the tears seemed to have receded. Another deep breath. I pressed my cold hands to my hot cheeks and stepped off the elevator, shoulders back, head up. I avoided direct eye contact. Marion's words marched through my mind, a ticker tape of syllables—*make all the arrangements now, make all the arrangements, now make all the arrangements, make the*— I rubbed my thumb along the smooth metal back of my phone. I knew the number for Queen's Park Cemetery, 403-221-3660. I'd looked it up in the phone book at the pay phones—*make the arrangements, now, 403-221-3660, make the...* At Queen's Park, where Cec's mother was buried. Cec had already said she wanted to be buried there, in the same plot as her parents, if possible. I wasn't sure it would be possible. Her father was buried in the veteran's section. Her mother had been cremated and an urn with her ashes had been buried alongside him.

Trevor, Cec's brother, had been cremated at Queen's Park, also Ellen, Cec's sister.

They had pulled Ellen's body out of the refrigerator when Cec had said she wanted to see her.

"You want a viewing?" The program director, a young guy in a grey suit, had looked perplexed.

"No, not a viewing." Lora was sitting across from Cec. I was beside her. Sheila, Cec's sister from Long Island, was there too.

"I don't want a formal viewing," Cec said. "I just want to see her."

We were sitting at a round table in a room with neutral decor designed to have a calming effect.

"I suppose we could. But it wouldn't be—I mean—she won't be made up." The program director was speaking toward Cec, but mostly to himself.

"Doesn't need to be formal," Cec said.

"It would be very informal." The program director sounded apologetic. "And you would have to understand, her colouration won't be normal. She may look slightly blue, especially around her eyes."

Cec nodded, the fire drained out of her.

"There'll be an additional charge."

"Whatever. I'll cover it."

He stood up. "I'll need a moment."

The program director left the room.

"I don't know if I can," Lora whispered, her voice even smaller than usual.

"I'll go with you." Sheila reached over and put her hand on Cec's arm.

"You don't have to. No one has to…" Cec's voice quavered. She just wanted to see her sister.

I understood. Viewing is part of the Mennonite tradition. I'd been looking at dead white faces since I was tall enough to stand on tiptoe and peer over the edge of a casket. It was okay to touch, to lay a warm hand on the cold one, to bend over and kiss the waxen forehead or cheek. Dead cheeks always looked so sunken and strangely angular. It made sense to me, even as a child, that the dead be put on display. Their unbreathing stillness offered a confirmation, a resounding testament, to the fact that the spirit had fled the body.

But Cec's family didn't understand how to arrange a viewing. They seemed to have no ritual around death at all. Cec said she'd never been to a funeral as a kid. Well, except one, sort of. Her uncle had died and she'd driven with her dad to Manitoba. But he hadn't let her go to the service.

When Cec's brother Trevor died, his body had been so emaciated that no one had any desire to view him.

Ellen was different. Her death was self-induced and unexplained. No note. There wouldn't be a casket.

The program director returned. "You can follow me," he said and pulled Cec's chair back as she stood up. I got up too, as did Sheila. Lora hesitated, then stood.

He led us to a back hallway and through a door to a long, narrow room with yellow walls. Along one wall there were rows of square, stainless-steel doors: three high, half a dozen across.

Cec had agreed to informal. But this?

Ellen was lying on a stainless-steel metal trolley that had been positioned against the wall across from the bank of doors. Her lips had been stitched shut, or maybe glued. Her eyeballs had sunk into her skull. A dark-blue blanket was pulled up to her collarbone. What looked like the ridges of her knuckles pushed the blanket up across her middle, fingers apparently folded together.

"Ell…" Cec's body sagged. I reached for her. One more step and she was beside Ellen, leaning against the trolley. "Oh, Ell…" Cec put her hand on top of the outline of Ellen's hands. I was at Ellen's feet. Sheila had stopped just inside the doorway. Lora hovered behind Sheila.

"I'm so sorry. So sorry," Cec bent forward until her face was right beside Ellen's, whispering, as she brushed Ellen's hair back from her forehead.

I turned to leave, to give Cec time alone with her, but Sheila and Lora had stepped into the room and were right behind me. I'd have to push past them and I didn't have the energy. I turned back to Ellen. Her forehead was a translucent bluish hue, a lighter blue at her temples. I couldn't help but wonder if the blue was from the antifreeze. They'd found an opened container of antifreeze on Ellen's kitchen counter and a mug on the floor with what looked like the remains of red wine.

Cec touched Ellen's face with her fingertips, "Oh, baby…" and then words I couldn't hear. Sheila and Lora were both beside me now. Sheila's eyes were closed, her lips moving.

I pushed myself up out of the hard-backed green chair at the end of Cec's bed. The chair legs scraped. I halted mid-rise to see whether the sound had woken Cec. Her tongue flicked between dry lips. She murmured but didn't open her eyes.

I walked quietly toward the door and out into the hall.

At a right angle to Cec's room, the door to the cleaning room stood open, a white plastic chair just inside. I sank into it. I didn't want Cec to see me take out my cellphone. I didn't want her to hear me. But I also didn't want to be too far away in case she needed me.

The receptionist who answered was polite, though her voice sounded tired. She forwarded me along. The next voice was cheerier and yes, she could help me. This was her area of expertise. I could tell by the way she said, "What is the name of the person for whom you are making the arrangements?"

"Cecile Kaysoe." And then my throat closed up. I squeezed my eyes shut. I couldn't believe I was making this call, about to have this conversation.

"Does she have pre-arrangements filed with us?"

"No."

"Does she have a will?"

"Yes."

"Are any of her wishes in writing?"

"Yes, but…I, uh…need to confirm…a few details."

"Do you know whether she would prefer cremation or burial?"

I got up out of the chair and paced. "Burial. I think." When we'd originally made our wills, Cec had said she wanted to be buried. But that was several years ago. "Let's say burial, for now."

"Of course…" I was leaning against the door jamb my head turned so I could see into Cec's room. "When can you come in?" She'd need my signature.

Cec's eyes opened. She turned and looked right at me. *Did she know what I was doing?* My heart pounding, I said I had to go and flipped my phone shut.

Cec gave me a long, blank stare as I walked back into the room. I hoped she hadn't heard. I tried to smile, but it was a weak effort.

Cec closed her eyes. She hadn't thrown up since the contents of her stomach had been pumped out. Morphine seemed to be numbing her pain. I watched her drift, and rouse, then drift again.

What was it I needed to say to her? Marion was right. I should say what I needed to say while she could still respond, if she wanted to.

I would tell her how much I loved her, but that was such a cliché.

I wanted to ask her about Christian. Or did I? Cec hadn't talked about him in a long time and it might be strange to bring him up again, out of nowhere.

I knew what I wouldn't tell her: that I'd wished her gone, more than once, when I was hurt and furious and blurry with tears.

Like that night when all the dogs had started barking, just after midnight, all of them at once. They'd sounded serious. We'd both scrambled out of bed to find all the cows grazing on the front lawn.

"Really?" Cec looked at me. "Again?"

"It wasn't me."

"Uh huh."

We hurried into chore clothes and Cec ran to the barn to get a pail of oats. She shook the pail, rattling the oats. The cows lifted their heads. They understood the sound of oats. They ambled toward her. She walked slowly toward the pasture gate with a trail of cows following. I shooed from behind.

As soon as the gate was closed and before she could launch another accusation, I said, "You were the last one out here last night."

"I closed it."

"You must not have."

"I know I did."

"This is *not* my fault!" I said.

She stood with her hands on her hips, head cocked.

"It's not!" I wasn't about to back down.

She stared at me expressionless. "What's your fault is your fault, and what's my fault is your fault."

Everything that was her fault was my fault? Was she kidding? I waited for some indication she was joking. Nothing.

She turned and walked toward the house. As I watched her walk away my outrage dissipated, slowly transforming into clarity: *I don't need to listen to anything she says.* She could zing me with her sharpest barbs, change the direction of her attack, deflect deflect deflect. It didn't matter.

I heard her open the back door, then slam it shut. I stood staring at the corrals swiping at the tears on my cheeks with the backs of my hands.

I was contemplating a possibility. It was inching closer.

Just me.

By myself.

Without her.

I waited until she opened her eyes. She seemed to be lucid.

I took her hand. I said, "I love you."

She looked at me blankly. I wondered whether she had heard me.

"I know," she said.

I let go of her hand. *Of course. What had I expected?* "Babe?"

"I told you not to call me that."

I let her words slide. "I need to go out to the farm," I said.

"Doreen's doing chores."

"I need to get our papers."

"Papers?"

"Registrations for the cars. Your will."

"Why?"

"We need to go through it all. And you need to sign the cars over to me."

"There's still time."

I wanted to say, *Really? How much?* What I said was, "I need to check on the dogs." I hadn't told her that I'd put the dogs in the kennel.

She didn't say anything. I think she could sense my determination.

"I thought this afternoon would be a good time. Kara is on. You like her."

Cec closed her eyes.

I waited. I leaned back in my chair, closed my eyes. Did I drift off? When I opened my eyes again she was looking at me.

"Go at four o'clock," she said. "That way you can get back before the night nurse comes on."

Kara was trying to convince Cec to take a stronger enema as I put on my jacket and gathered myself to leave.

Cec was shaking her head. She looked at me and said, "Tell her."

"She knows," I said, as gently as I could.

"I'll bring it and you can decide." Kara left the room and returned with a jug of clear liquid. It was the same shape and size as a jug of windshield-washer fluid. The label said GoLightly.

"All of that?!" Cec shook her head. "There's no way!"

"As much as you can."

I hesitated. Maybe this wasn't a good time to go.

"Only a little." Cec showed Kara what she meant with her thumb and forefinger.

"More than that. As much as you can."

"I'll be back soon," I said to Cec.

"You're going?"

"I need to check on the dogs. Remember? It's four o'clock."

"You have to go now?"

I wondered whether I should stay. But I needed to go. Kara was with her. She would be okay. "I won't be long."

I drove quickly, amazed at the quiet light on the prairie and how much the snow had melted. How many days had she been in the hospital? Five? Six. Seven. I hadn't been out to the farm for a week.

Spring calves were starting to appear in the pastures. The farther I drove, the lighter I felt. I had made good on a much-needed escape. Cec was in competent hands. I could let myself relax for a couple of hours, appreciate the wide expanse of open sky, breathe in the fresh air. I called Doreen on my way out and told her that I was on my way home and would take care of chores.

I didn't remember until I turned onto the driveway that the cows were gone. No boney rumps lined up for feed. All that remained were scrape marks across the corral where Hank and Jake had dragged the panels to trap the cows and force them up the shoot. They'd even managed to get Sham into the trailer. Doreen said he hadn't put up much of a fight. And she had taken Griff and Charlie to the kennel. I missed their exuberant welcome, but it was better they weren't here.

I gave the horses, llamas, goats, and chickens extra feed and made sure they all had fresh water. It felt familiar, and also foreign, to be walking on clumps of melting snow listening to the grunts of the animals.

I should have worked faster. A prick of urgency nudged me to hurry but I ignored it. Lugging bales was restorative. I needed restoration.

When the animals were all fed, I went into the house

and collected the pile of bills from Cec's desk. I pulled open the top drawer of her filing cabinet and found a file folder labeled CECILE – WILL. I opened the folder to double-check. Yes, there was the original.

In another folder I found the registrations for the cars. My car was registered in my name but all the other vehicles—her car, the half-ton, the van—were registered in hers.

Her first instinct was always to pay. It was never a question. She reached for her wallet, never flinched at the amount, made picking up the tab look effortless. I paid the mortgage. She took care of everything else. It worked best that way.

I opened the second drawer of her filing cabinet. No file folders, just a pile of unopened letters from the CRA. *She hadn't opened any of them?* The envelopes filled the drawer. *What did the CRA want with Cec? What hadn't she told me?* I picked up one of the envelopes. I would take it with me, get Cec to open it or tell me what was in it. *Maybe I should just open it. No, I'd rather she tell me.*

I got back on the road later than I'd intended and felt a twinge of guilt. Kara would be gone by the time I got there. The night nurse would have started. I hadn't checked who it was. Even when it was one of the good ones they had to do a complete round at the beginning and sometimes Cec's morphine was delayed.

I ran across the parking lot and racewalked down the hall.

I should have run.

Her room was dark. Cec was sitting in one of the high-back chairs, no housecoat, no slippers, hands gripping the armrests, jaw clenched, face as white as her nightie.

Shit!

"Get someone!" she hissed at me. "I can't do this anymore."

"Hang on, Babe!"

Who had let this happen?

I ran down the hall to the nurses' station and checked the board. Nadine was her assigned. *Oh great, a new one.*

"Where's Nadine?" I said in the direction of the nurses' station.

"That's me." She was leaning against the counter at the nurses' station.

"Cecile is in extreme pain. Room 13."

"Because of the GoLightly," she said, entirely unconcerned.

"What is that stuff?"

If anyone had told me what GoLightly does inside the body, I would never have let them give it to Cec. It draws fluid from all other parts of the body into the bowels. The resulting pressure was beyond what Cecile should ever have been asked to bear.

Nadine followed me back to the room and stood in front of Cec, her hands on her hips. "Is the pain still bad?"

"I can't *dooo* this—"

"She can't do this anymore!" *Was this woman stupid? What part of extreme pain did she not comprehend?* "We need to hook her up to the stomach pump again." I tried to keep my voice even. "Get that stuff out of her stomach."

"Only if a resident gives the order."

"Then get a resident in here!"

"I cannn't…" From Cec.

Nadine left the room. I crouched in front of Cec and said, "I'll find someone. I will *not* let them leave you like this. I'll be right back."

She didn't respond, her jaw clenched, her neck straining.

I ran to the nurses' station. Nadine could go to hell!

"Who's in charge?" I asked the woman behind the desk.

"Melinda," she said, turning around, pointing toward the back office. Melinda emerged wearing a smock covered in teddy bears. "Is there a problem?"

I nodded. "Cecile is not being properly attended. Come with me." I spoke with as much calm and determination as I could muster. I knew that my urgency had the potential to erupt and I couldn't afford to let it.

"Who is her assigned?"

"Nadine. She's gone to call the resident. We need to hook Cec back up to the stomach pump. She was given GoLightly. Her pain is unbearable. She's being steamrolled." My words tumbled over themselves.

Melinda followed me to Cec's room. We passed Nadine in the hallway. She glared at me. I said nothing and, surprisingly, Melinda didn't either.

Melinda was reluctant to hook Cec back up to the stomach pump, said she would need an order from a resident.

"But why? The resident gave the order before. Isn't that enough?"

"She's been given GoLightly. We need to give it a chance to work."

"But she can't stand it."

"I cannn't," Cec was pleading.

"Can you call the resident? Get permission over the phone?"

"I can try, but can't guarantee anything. I could increase her morphine."

"Fentanyl," Cec said.

"They switched you?" I asked.

Cec nodded.

"She'll probably be more comfortable in her bed," Melinda said.

"Recliner." Cec motioned to the pink vinyl recliner.

Melinda helped me move Cec. I got another blanket from the cart in the hallway and asked Melinda for a hot-water bottle, but Cec shook her head, no, she didn't want that.

Cec was breathing fast and hard. Melinda said she'd ask

about increasing her Fentanyl.

What I was about to learn the hard way was that the shift to a new NSAID (non-steroidal anti-inflammatory drug) is not an exact science. The right level of medication is a matter of trial and error. Some people respond more sensitively to some narcotics than others. Some respond better to certain types.

As it turned out, Cec had not responded well to Fentanyl. She needed a much higher dose than she'd been given and Nadine hadn't been paying attention. Kara would have been able to tell immediately, instinctively. Sanjay said later there was also a possibility that Cec had had an allergic reaction.

Melinda left to call the resident and Cec gripped my hand so hard I thought she would crush a bone. I didn't object. My pain was a mere fraction of hers.

"I'll give her one minute, then I'll go see if she got the order."

Cec sat with her eyes closed, moving her head back and forth, groaning.

"I'm so sorry. So sorry." *Was there any atonement sufficient?*

I counted out sixty seconds. I said to Cec, "I'm going to go see if she's talked with the resident."

Nothing from Cec.

"I'll be back really soon."

I extricated my hand from her grasp and walked, almost jogged, to the nurses' station.

Melinda had talked with the resident on call. He said he wanted to examine Cecile before they hooked her back up to the stomach pump.

"When is he coming?

"As soon as he can."

I knew exactly how long it could take for a resident to appear—all night, or longer.

"And this," I bent down so I was eye to eye with Melinda, "is the best we can do for her? She's in extreme distress. Did you tell him?"

"I told him."

"Will that get him here any faster?"

"He said he'd come as soon as he could."

"We both know what that means."

She knew, and to her credit, she looked sheepish.

I said, "If he's not here in five minutes, I'm going to hook her up to the pump myself."

"I would strongly advise against that."

"I'll be happy to let you do it. But if you don't, or won't, then I will."

"You don't know how. You could hurt her."

"There is no possible way I could inflict anymore pain on her than she's in right now." I started back down the hall.

"If he's not here in fifteen minutes," Melinda called after me, "I'll hook her up."

"Five!" I said over my shoulder. "And thank you."

When I got back to the room, I said, "They've called the resident. If he's not here in five minutes, they'll hook you up again."

Through clenched teeth, Cec said, "I have a…pain… in my chest."

"You do?"

She nodded. "Tell them." She motioned with her chin in the direction of the CALL button.

God, she was bright! Even in this kind of pain, she had the wherewithal to play her trump card.

"They have no idea who they're dealing with, do they?" If I hadn't been so tight with fury I would have started laughing.

"Sick of this!" she said.

No kidding. I was too. I hit the CALL button, "Cecile has a pain in her chest."

"Hello?" from the other end. "Repeat please."

"Cecile has a pain in her chest. Hurry!" I used my best

panic voice.

Immediate action. Nurses running down the hall.

Cec gave me a grim smile. Her expression said: *See! That's how you do it!* Narcotics hadn't dulled her genius for getting others to do her bidding.

Two nurses burst into the room, stethoscopes at the ready. One took her blood pressure. A resident had been called and would be coming immediately. An EKG machine was on its way.

Cec didn't have to fake her pain, just the location. She was happy to oblige the nurses with breathless one- and two-word answers. But I don't think she'd counted on having to lie flat on her back for an EKG (electrocardiogram). The nurses were insistent. It would only take a minute. But I knew it wasn't the length of time that mattered. Even a single second on her back would exponentially intensify the pain.

The resident was a tall, slender woman with long dark hair. She brought a measure of humanity with her competence. Why couldn't Cec have been assigned to this woman rather than the impressed-with-himself Steader?

I don't remember the resident's name. What I remember is that her fingernails were painted deep purple and she was wearing three-inch red heels. She didn't ask Cec whether she wanted an EKG. She had the nurses roll the machine into the room and instructed them to get Cec positioned.

I said, "It hurts her to lie flat." These people had no idea.

"It would be best if you waited in the hall."

A small part of me wanted to stay with Cec, but mostly I didn't.

A nurse nudged me out of the room. I heard Cec moan, then yell, "AAAAAHHHH..." I sat down in an empty wheelchair. Cec cried out again. I heard a murmur of voices and the rolling of wheels on the industrial-grade lino.

I was allowed back into the room after the EKG machine was gone. Cec was in bed, the back raised.

"Can't do this anymore," I heard Cec whisper.

The resident was standing at Cec's bedside, her back to me. "You're not having a heart attack, that's the good news."

"Can't!" Cec's cheeks were flushed.

"The best way to stop the pain will be to knock you out with sleeping pills."

"No pills." Cec became agitated. "Tell her!" Cec said to me.

The resident turned to me.

"She doesn't like sleeping pills. Is there another way?"

"It's the best way. She needs a rest."

"What about hooking her back up to the stomach pump?"

"It's been about five hours since she was given the enema. At this point pumping her stomach won't provide any significant relief."

"Put me out. For good," Cec said.

I knew what she was asking.

The resident said, "I can give you two different sleeping pills to make sure you're knocked out."

"Don't want sleeping pills. I want this over. For good."

The resident didn't answer for a moment. Then she said, "If I could, legally, I would help you. The best I can do is knock you out."

"What about increasing the Fentanyl?" I asked.

"She's already at the max."

"Could you switch her to something else?"

"It would be best to keep her on Fentanyl for a while. Give the morphine a chance to clear out of her system."

The resident and I both looked at Cec. She was shaking her head, no.

"Cec, I think you should let her give you the sleeping pills."

"I thought you were on my side."

"I am. You need to sleep."

"I would give you an Ativan," the resident said to Cec,

"and a T—" the name flew by too fast. "The Ativan is longer acting and the other is short term. The two together should ensure that you sleep for more than just a couple of hours."

Cec shook her head. "I don't know."

"I'll be here," I said, and reached for her hand.

She waved my hand away. "I can't make any more decisions." She looked defeated.

The resident looked at me and raised her eyebrows.

I nodded, yes.

"I'll have the nurse bring the pills."

"How long will she be out?"

"Six to eight hours." She turned and left the room.

Cecile said to me, "She's no good."

"She's doing what she can."

"Do you have the stuff?"

"The stuff?"

"Plan B. I told you to get the stuff. It's time."

"No. I don't." I felt nauseated and overwhelmingly inadequate. I knew I was letting her down. All I could say, in a whisper like a confession, was, "I had no idea it would be today. How could I know that?"

"There's a Swiss Army knife in my purse. Leave it beside the sink in the bathroom. I'll take care of it."

My thoughts went to the unused prescription painkillers in her purse, Naproxen and OxyContin. But since she hadn't been able to hold anything down, they were probably no longer an option.

Nadine brought two small pills and a cup of water.

"Here goes nothing," Cec said. "Where's the basin? These might come back." She swallowed.

I waited, basin at the ready. The pills stayed down.

"Would you like another blanket?"

She shook her head, no. Her eyes closed. I let myself imagine that the pills were a lethal dose of something. That's all it would take, and this could all be over. I wouldn't say a word. No one would be culpable.

Cec looked like she was sleeping.

I leaned close and whispered, "Cec?"

She didn't respond. I squeezed her hand. Nothing. I sank into the recliner and leaned back. The tremors of fury were subsiding, fatigue beginning to take hold.

A nurse I didn't know, not Nadine, came into the room pushing a fold-up cot on wheels. "So you can stay with her," she said. She moved several of the visitors' chairs out into the hall to make room for the cot and positioned it along the wall at the end of Cec's bed.

"Thank you," I whispered. Cec's eyes still hadn't opened. The nurse left and I sat, tears running. I didn't know why I was crying. Most likely because Cec was finally asleep and couldn't see me.

The nurse was back, with blankets and a pillow.

"I really appreciate this," I said, blowing my nose, "but I'm going to go to my parents' for the night."

"I'll leave them for you anyway. You might need them another time."

I rummaged through Cec's bag. I found her Swiss Army knife and put it in my purse. I wasn't entirely sure, but I thought there was a pretty good chance that if she killed herself, I wouldn't get the life insurance. I felt guilty for being so selfish, but that's what I was thinking as I looked for her tweezers, and nail clippers, and anything else that she might use to slice her wrists.

I knew that Cec wasn't considering the possible impact of her actions on me. She wasn't thinking coherently much of the time. But I was relatively confident she would understand. I didn't want to be left with nothing at the end of this. She wouldn't want that for me either.

Before I left, I stood at Cec's bedside. I wanted to make sure she was really out. I knew that she was often still aware, even when her eyes were closed. This time her breathing was deeper. Her eyelids flickered.

"Cec," I whispered and touched her hand.

No response.

"I'm going now."

Not a twitch.

"I'll be back first thing in the morning."

Nothing.

I fell into an uneasy sleep at Mom and Dad's, closed my eyes to the shadowy walls. I dreamed that I was lying on the cot in Cec's hospital room, facing the wall, my body curled tight as a fist, clothes still on. I heard a groan. At first I thought the sound was coming from me. I opened my eyes. All I could make out were dark, shadowy shapes. I stood up, swaying, bare feet on the cold tile floor, and felt my way around Cec's bed toward the door. Cec groaned again. I stopped. Her breathing resumed.

I tried to open the wide steel door leading out into the hallway. It was locked. Locked? I jiggled the handle. I yanked. Nothing. I opened my mouth to yell but the sound stuck in my throat. The CALL button glowed red on Cec's bedside table and as I reached to push it, the door to Cec's room swung open, as if on some kind of command.

I stepped into the bright hospital hallway, except that I wasn't walking, I was floating under flickering fluorescent lights. The hallway was lined with beds: a wooden bunk bed with disheveled blue blankets covered in red fire trucks; a double bed neatly made up with a pristine white duvet; a waterbed without covers, just the mattress, sloshing; an empty hospital bed with hospital-issue blankets pushed aside, the impression of a body still fresh; a bed with a red canopy and a quilt of deep red covered in gold leaves.

A man in a black trench coat was lying on the red-canopied bed, his black leather shoes still on.

"Tell your shoes to be quiet." I said.

"They're as quiet at they can be." His voice was deep, resonant.

He opened his trench coat. I lay down beside him, inside his coat. He wrapped his arms and his coat around me.

"I know about the dogs," he said.

Relief rippled through me. I wouldn't have to tell Cec.

I wondered, fleetingly, whether he was an assassin. It didn't matter. His trench coat smelled of damp dirt.

I wouldn't tell Cec that I had found comfort in the arms of a man.

Or that I spent most of Anna's wedding reception in the bathroom because I couldn't bear the way she smiled at her new husband with shy, happy eyes.

This man knew. His body heat warmed me through.

"She needs me," I said, lifting my face.

He opened his trench coat.

I lifted up into the air, hovering just above him.

The night before Anna's wedding, I leaned in close to a bathroom mirror as I drew a moustache on my upper lip with black water-soluble marker. I had been assured that the ink would wash off. I hoped it would. I stepped back from the mirror for a critical appraisal. A small group of women, mostly in their teens and twenties, were crowded into the bathroom trying to paint on their own moustaches, attach false beards. Once we had transformed ourselves into male facsimiles, we would descend upon Anna, dress her up in an old-fashioned flower-print dress with a lace collar, rouge her lips, add a grey wig, and parade her along the main walking street in Herning.

I pulled on a thrift-store tweed jacket and a battered fedora, a turquoise tie. I went to see whether I could get another moment in front of the mirror. The moustache was insufficient. I leaned in close to the mirror and blackened my chin, surprised at how easily a painted-on beard transformed my face. I found it a bit unnerving to see a dark-haired, young man staring back at me. Convincingly male, I thought, with that square-ish Mennonite angle to my chin.

I didn't want to be a man. But if I could have, I would have put on a tux and taken Kent's place at the altar the next morning. I would have been the one waiting for Anna in my shined shoes and boutonniere at the front of the church. I would have been the one she kissed when the reception guests tinkled their glasses, the one she smiled at shyly, the one who undid the hundred buttons down the back of her wedding dress at the end of the day.

I wasn't that guy. I would never be that guy. I was a young woman in an old man's fedora and a tweed jacket fumbling awkwardly, self-consciously, with my tie.

Wednesday, March 9

Lorraine stopped me in the hallway just as I was about to push open the door.

"I was hoping I'd catch you," she said, breathless. "Before you go in there, there's something you need to know."

My heart rate accelerated.

"She woke up. Just after you left last night. She was hallucinating and determined to leave. She ripped out her IV and pulled out her stomach tube. She looks pretty beat up. I didn't want you to walk in there without knowing."

"How is she now?"

"Incoherent. She still wants to leave. Someone has been with her all night."

"You should have called me."

"You needed to sleep."

"What am I supposed to do?"

"Let her know you're here. But be prepared, she may not know who you are. And," I felt the light touch of her hand on my arm, "they've had to restrain her."

"Tie her down?"

"Her hands and feet, and a body jacket. For her safety."

I couldn't tell which was greater, my rage at myself that I'd left last night, or terror at the thought of pushing open her door.

I didn't want to go in there.

I stood with my hand pressed flat on the cool steel and thought about turning around, walking back down the hall.

I pushed open the door.

The curtain was pulled back. The back of Cec's bed had been lowered. Didn't they know she couldn't lie flat?

Cec had raised herself up onto her elbows. Her face was puffy, flushed. One side of her face, under her right eye, was bruised. Deep blue. Crusted blood around her nostrils, spatters of blood on her hands and arms, smears on her hospital nightie. A jagged welt, red, blue, and puffy, gaped open on the back of her right hand.

"Lemme go! I hafta go!" Her voice was hoarse but commanding, directed at the two attendants, a young man and a young woman, both in white lab coats. They were standing on the far side of the bed, recruited to stand sentry. The way they looked up at me, with hope and expectation, I could see they wanted to bolt.

Cec's wrists were bound with bands of white cloth tied to the bed frame. The tie-downs were long enough that she could move her hands. She was waving a clenched fist.

This was not Cecile. This was…she was…

She turned to me, her eyes wild. "You have to get me out of here," she growled, her voice deep, gravelly.

"I can't, Babe." I was speaking from somewhere outside of me. "The doctors won't let me." I had no idea where the words were coming from.

Her voice sank lower, as if from some netherworld: "What kind of hold do they have on you?!"

"You have to work with me." I crouched down so I was eye level with her. I spoke softly, conspiratorially. "First, we need to get your pain under control." I had no idea whether she was in any pain. She seemed to relax, just a bit. "Then we'll talk with the doctors." I tried to sound as though I had some sort of authority.

Cec pulled at her body jacket with both hands, yanking at the white cloth bound tightly round her torso. Her movements were determined but uncoordinated.

"Maybe we should untie her." The young male attendant took hold of her wrist and undid the knot.

I reached toward him, panicked. "I'm not sure that's a good idea." But he had already freed one of her arms and Cec was now helping him to untie the other. The female attendant was undoing the ties around her ankles.

They were going to cut her loose and leave me alone with her.

Cec grinned at me, a maniacally triumphant grin.

The young man crawled under the bed to untie the body jacket. As the jacket loosened, Cec sat up straighter. She pulled her rings from her fingers. She wore two rings, one on the fourth finger of each hand. The gold band was from me. The other, a tiny diamond solitaire, had been a gift from a guy she'd had an affair with while she was still married to Jens. She handed me her rings. I took them.

Arms free, she struggled to get out of the body jacket. She beat back the assistance of the young man. I wondered, as I watched, how they'd ever got her into the straitjacket in the first place. There must have been a small army.

As soon as she was free, Cec flung her legs over the side of the bed. Flapping her arms, she beat back the young female and stumbled around the bed.

I stepped in front of her to block her progress.

She slowed.

I grabbed hold of her shoulders.

She stopped.

I said, "We have to get your pain under control, remember? You need to work with me so we can get you out of here."

She took two steps toward the recliner and sat down, closed her eyes. Her head fell sideways, her mouth opened.

"Could someone please get me a blanket?"

The young woman had made a hurried exit but the young man was still a few steps from the door. He nodded.

I couldn't leave her. Not for a moment. Ever again. I'd

left her last night and that had been a mistake. I should have stayed. She would have recognized my voice. She would have felt less desperate.

I covered her with the blanket. Her feet were icy. I found her slippers and pulled them onto her swollen feet. "I'm so sorry..." I didn't know whether she could hear me. "I should have been here."

Cec lifted her head, opened her eyes, and lurched up out of the recliner in one swift motion.

"Hafta outta 'ere," she muttered, two steps ahead of me. I hurried to catch up and grabbed hold of her arm.

"Hang on. We need to wait for the doctor."

"Got go! Out this!" She yanked her arm out of my hand with surprising strength and got ahead of me again and out the door. I caught up, took hold of her arm, more firmly this time.

"Hey! Wait! We need to go back to the room." I was walking quickly, almost jogging to keep up. One of her slippers came off. She didn't slow down.

Lorraine appeared from an adjacent room. She grabbed hold of Cec's other arm.

"Going!" Cec said, emphatically, but then stopped. Lorraine gave her a gentle push and knocked her off balance in the direction of a wheelchair. She stumbled and we lowered her into a wheelchair. Her head fell back. Her eyes closed.

"She's pretty determined."

Lorraine set Cec's feet into the footrests and wheeled her back into her room. She seemed to be sleeping.

I used my shoulder to hold my cellphone against my ear. I called Lora. "She's delirious. You need to come." My voice was hushed.

"Delirious?"

"Incoherent. She's sleeping now but when she wakes up she tries to run. She wants to go home."

"Don't blame her."

"She needs people around her that she knows."

Lorraine had pushed Cec in the wheelchair into the room, and positioned it close to Cec's bed. I was standing behind the wheelchair so that Cec's head could rest against my belly. I ran my fingers through her hair as I dialed with my thumb.

"Hi, Mom."

"Lynnie, what's wrong?"

"She's delirious."

"What?!"

"She ripped out her IV and her stomach tube."

"Oh no. Do you want me to come?"

"Yes."

Cec opened her eyes. "Wee fluff," she said.

"I have to go—"

She got up out of the wheelchair, but I was ready for her. I had hold of both her forearms before she had taken her second step. She looked at me blankly.

"You need to sit down."

She didn't move.

"The doctors are going to come and you need to be here so we can talk with them."

She shook her head, an almost imperceptible no.

"How about the green chair?" I loosened my grip. She kept her eyes on my face as she shuffled sideways toward the green visitor's chair. She sat down.

"Are you cold?" I picked up a blanket and tucked it around her legs. Her eyes closed again.

"Sheed one."

"What did you say?"

"Feed lot outta this." The syllables were slurred. She waved her hand vaguely in my direction, eyes still closed.

Lorraine came into the room. "How is she?"

"I don't know." I was sitting beside Cec, my hand on her arm, sticking close in case she decided to bolt again.

"Would she like a Popsicle?"

"Ask her."

Lorraine tapped Cec's shoulder. Cec opened her eyes.

"Would you like a Popsicle?"

Cec nodded.

"What colour?"

"Orange."

"Orange? You don't like orange, remember?" I smiled, happy to hear a word that made some kind of lopsided sense.

Cec waved her hand. "Feed it to the rabbits."

"Well, let's try orange," I said. But when Lorraine brought an orange Popsicle Cec pushed it away.

"Okay, blue it is."

Cec accepted the blue Popsicle and held the wooden stick loosely between thumb and forefinger.

"It's going to melt." I nudged the dripping Popsicle toward her lips. She leaned the tip against her upper lip, took one small lick with her tongue. A blue drop fell onto the front of her white nightie, then another. Wet blue surrounded her lips and stained her tongue.

"Should I take it?" Blue was dripping down her hand and onto her lap. She shook her head and jerked the Popsicle out of my reach.

"Get her! The woman in the skirt!" Cec shook her finger emphatically at Lorraine.

"Cecile? Do you know where you are?"

"Under the desk."

"I think we should dial her down." Lorraine checked the IV monitor.

"Yes!" An exaggerated head bob from Cec. "She has it now!" Cec sat up, pointing.

"Who has it?"

"The woman!"

"Cecile, I'm Lorraine. I'm your nurse."

Lora was crouched beside Cec, her hand on Cec's arm. We were taking turns playing watchdog.

Lorraine had confirmed that Cec's appointment at the cancer centre had been cancelled. They had an opening on the fourteenth but we'd have to wait and see.

"Do you think she'll come back?" I asked Lorraine. Not that I expected her to know.

"You really want her to."

"Yes, I do."

"Then I hope she does." Lorraine squeezed my arm as she left to finish her rounds.

Lora looked up at me to say something. At that moment Cec bolted, up and out of the chair. She got ahead of us before we were fully mobilized. She strode determinedly, pumping her arms. It took both of us, one at each elbow, to slow her down. For someone who had been unable to walk to the bathroom unaided just twelve hours ago, she was miraculously strong.

Then her burst of determination flamed out and she sank into one of the vinyl recliners that lined the hallway.

"She sure knows how to boogie!" Lora was breathless.

"Is she okay?" Mom had just arrived and was standing behind me. Cec's eyes were closed.

"Yeah, she's okay. We'll just roll her back to her room."

"How often has she done this?" Mom asked.

"A few times. She's pretty serious about getting out of here," I released the wheels of the recliner and pushed Cec back down the hall.

I asked Lora to remove the recliner that was in Cec's room so I could roll her in. I tilted Cec back and swaddled her legs in blankets, tucked the sides in firmly around her. She would have to work to wriggle free.

In my dream I am walking down the hospital hallway and Cec comes out of her room to meet me. She is barefoot, in her white hospital gown with tiny blue flowers. Her cheeks are rosy, legs solid and strong, hair freshly washed and blown dry.

She smiles when she sees me and opens her arms for a hug.

We stand in the hallway and talk like old friends. We laugh at the ridiculousness of hospital gowns and the drips of blue Popsicle down her front.

She says that one day we will come back to this hallway. We'll remember these days. We'll talk about this moment.

Then she looks down at her bare feet and says, "I think you should bring the car around."

The door swung open. Sanjay, the tall, dark-skinned palliative doctor, with another doctor.

"Should I leave?" Mom asked.

"No. Stay."

"Hello," Dr. Sanjay nodded at me, Mom, and Lora in turn. "I'm Dr. Sanjay. This is Dr. Choy." Dr. Choy's thick black hair was poker straight and cut around his ears. The frames of his glasses were perfect circles, which gave his flat face the look of a precocious young boy.

Cec seemed to be sleeping and didn't stir at the doctors' arrival. Neither Sanjay nor Choy said anything to Cec or asked how she was doing. I sensed they had been fully briefed and knew she was still incoherent.

Sanjay flipped through the pages on his clipboard. His expression was sombre. "You wanted to know about prognosis," he said, without looking up. I hoped Marion had been stern with him. "The cancer is advanced. Stage four."

"We know."

"And aggressive."

This wasn't news.

"When cancer is advanced, as in this case, the end can come at any time." He lifted his hand flat, palm down, as though demonstrating the height of a small child. "She might go along and even seem to be doing fairly well," he moved his hand through the air along a straight line, "and then all of a sudden…" He dropped his hand, moving downward, a rollercoaster on the downslope. "Just like that, she could be gone."

"What does that mean? Days? Hours?"

"A lot depends on her, on her will. It could be a few days, or a week, or longer."

I wanted to ask him why he hadn't had the decency to tell us this before, when she was still coherent.

"The delirium…" I struggled to keep my voice steady. "Why did it happen?"

He flipped to another page on his clipboard. "There are five different factors that can contribute to a delirium. Four of the five were present in this case." He counted them off, lifting his fingers one by one: "Extreme pain. High calcium levels. Change in pain meds. Bladder infection."

"Bladder infection?"

"It showed up positive in the labs. We'll give her antibiotics and catheterize. And we'll take her off Fentanyl in case she's had a negative reaction, put her back on Hydromorph. We'll also put her on Haldol, an antipsychotic, which should help her to relax, and alleviate the hallucinations."

I looked at Choy, wondering why he had come.

"Will she come back?"

Sanjay hesitated. Choy took a half-step forward and said, "When cancer is this advanced, a delirium can be the beginning of the slippery slope."

"We asked you for a prognosis." I looked at Sanjay, who looked down at his clipboard. Choy's eyes met mine. "When she wasn't delirious." A quaver crept into my voice. I swallowed hard. *No tears. Not now.* "You told us," I turned to Sanjay, "that we'd have to wait and talk to the gyne-oncologist. At the cancer centre." Sanjay still wouldn't look at me. "You could have told us this," I brought my hand up, palm flat, then dropped it, "when she was coherent."

"The oncologist—" he said, but I cut him off.

"I want…" With all the strength I could summon, I said, "I want her to come back to me one more time."

Sanjay began scribbling on his clipboard as though these were instructions he needed to remember.

"That's what I want." I glared at each of them in turn. "I mean this."

I sat squeezing Cec's hand, inviting her to come back. I imagined the warmth of my touch as a small, bright light. Could she hear me calling out to her? *You don't have to stay long, but please come back.*

Her eyes opened. "Garfeel sheela wash car ring."

I leaned closer. "What?" As though I should be able to understand.

"Shir alun uppa skree." She lifted her hand and fluttered her fingers. The same fluttering movement through the air that her mother had made with her bent arthritic fingers. The wave of bird wings flapping. A bare flutter at eye level. Fluttering fingers moving away. Always away.

"Kadon radjish," she said emphatically, then, "my fall step…" trailing into unintelligible syllables.

"Are you in pain?"

She looked at me solemnly and shook her head, no.

She'd been without pain meds for almost twelve hours. I kept asking Lorraine whether we should give her Hydromorph, but Lorraine kept saying no, not as long as she wasn't in pain.

I closed my eyes as I tried to keep her pain at bay with the sheer stubbornness of my will. At some point the pain would rear up again. I'd seen it happen. She would be steamrolled. The nurses called it snowballing. The pain would crush her.

Steader stood quietly at Cec's bedside. She looked like she was sleeping. I said, in a low voice, "She had a bladder infection."

"Yes, she did."

"Her pain was out of control."

He didn't say anything. I think he could hear the anger in my voice.

"Her pain has not been well managed. That needs to change."

He nodded.

"I don't want this to happen again."

"We'll do our best."

Later, when I told Marion, she said, "You think he got it?"

"I'm pretty sure he did."

In a conversation I had with Marion after Cec was gone, she said to me, "Dr. Steader should have signed her over to palliative care."

"I thought he did."

"He consulted with palliative but he should have handed her care completely over to them. She would have had better pain management."

"That was his decision? Shouldn't it have happened automatically, her being signed over?"

"It's not automatic."

"No one ever said anything."

"Maybe I shouldn't have told you."

"I knew he was an egomaniac!"

"It wouldn't have changed the outcome."

"No, but if her pain could have been better managed…"

"Possibly, but maybe not."

"Will you put another IV in?" I asked Sanjay that evening. Choy was with him.

Sanjay hesitated, then said, "Might not be a good idea. In case she has another episode."

"It's hard to find a good vein." Lorraine had followed

the doctors into the room.

"We could go to a butterfly," Choy said.

"What's that?"

"It's a subcutaneous injection that's given manually."

Subcutaneous. I knew that word. From the instructions on bottles of tetracycline, an antibiotic that we'd had to give the calves. The trick was to get hold of a good handful of the hide between their shoulder blades, pull up, then jab the needle in under the skin but not into bone.

"It wouldn't go right into her bloodstream."

"No. But we need an injection site that she can't reach."

"How about her upper back, just above the shoulder blade? She couldn't reach it there," Lorraine suggested. She saw my quizzical look and said, "The butterfly is like the tip of a needle embedded in the skin. We insert it, tape it down, leave it there, so we don't need to poke her every time."

Sanjay seemed to think this was a good idea. He made a note.

Choy said, "You may want to call the family." He nodded solemnly, and with what felt like respect. "It's time."

Cec said once that she had never loved anyone like she loved me. She said it with a shake of her head as though she hoped to snap herself out of it. I could tell she wanted me to say the same back to her. I couldn't. She wasn't that person for me. I could have lied but she would have known.

So what I said, rather lamely, was, "Why me?"

She'd shrugged.

"What is it about me?" There was something about her, something that drew me, that held me in her orbit. You can't conjure attraction, or rationalize desire. It was there for me, but more about the physical, the sexual—more animal and less emotionally consuming I think, than it was for her.

"I don't know," her voice louder, irritated.

"Was it the—?"

"It just *is*, Lyn! It is what it is."

Cec's eyes were open, a vacant stare. It was easy for Lora, Mom, and I to talk around her. But I was determined to treat her like a regular person, include her in our conversation. I insisted that the nurses address their questions to her directly.

"Are you cold?" I asked her for the umpteenth time.

Cec shook her head, no.

"Are you hungry?"

Again, no.

"Are you in pain?"

She shook her head.

It was hard to know whether she really understood or whether her responses came from some deeper instinct. She showed no irritation. This, to me, was the greatest indication that the Cecile I knew was holed away inside a cave of psychosis. When she became irritated with my pestering, I'd know she was back.

"Noddy wants to come into our bedroom at night, oh yes, he does," my mother was saying to Lora. "I make a nice bed for him on the couch and I think he sleeps there but I'm not sure. We close our bedroom door. In the morning he's standing at the door waiting for us."

"He doesn't scratch?" Lora asked.

"No, he's very quiet."

Noddy must know, I thought. He's being good. I felt a pang of dog guilt. I'd seen so little of him. Mom and Dad had already had him for over a week and they weren't really keen on dogs.

"He's always happy to see us when we open the door. Richard takes him for a walk."

I watched Cec's face for any flicker of recognition at the mention of Noddy's name. She stared at Mom blankly, as if her mind had been scrubbed clean, or (and I shuddered at this thought) as if she'd been lobotomized.

"I wish we could let him out in the yard to pee, but we're missing a gate so the yard isn't completely enclosed. And besides, I've heard that dog pee kills the grass."

Lora said, "I've heard that too."

"Really?" I wasn't actually sure that was true. "We have three dogs. They all pee on our grass, and we only have a couple of dead spots. I'm not even sure the dead spots are from dog pee."

Cec would know this. I squeezed her arm, "Hey Cec, does dog pee kill grass?"

All three of us turned to her without expectation.

"Only females," Cec said.

"Only females?" That sounded like a coherent answer. I had to verify, "Only the pee from female dogs kills the grass?"

Cec nodded, her eyes still vacant.

"But our dogs are male and we still have dead spots on our lawn."

"Charlie," she said.

"Of course." Charlie was a female. I looked at Mom and Lora then turned to ask Cec another question but her eyes were closed.

"That sounded coherent," Mom said.

"It did."

Cec was still in there, somewhere.

Lora stepped out for a smoke. Mom left to do an errand. I was leaning back in the vinyl recliner, blankets bunched against my back. I didn't have the energy to rearrange them. Cec was in her bed in her almost-sitting position and didn't seem to be in pain. Still no painkillers. I was becoming increasingly uncomfortable with this calm. Somewhere inside Cec's body, mutinous cells were building blockages.

When Mom returned she had a magazine and a book. She said that she could sit in the hallway if that was better.

"No. Come in here. Please. Could you stay with her for a couple of hours?" I was determined that Cec would never be left alone again. "I'd like to go to your place and have a shower, maybe even have a nap."

"Take as long as you need."

I was back two hours later, after a shower and a half hour of lying on Mom and Dad's guest bed staring at the ceiling.

When I walked into the room, Cec was sitting up in bed.

Sitting up?

She turned to me when I walked into the room but kept on talking to Mom just as though this was any other afternoon in Room 13, in Ward 51. "One of her books. The first one, I think." Cec's speech was slow but her eyes were bright.

Mom was holding *Traveling Mercies* by Anne Lamott. "She's a minister?" Mom asked.

"Not in a church."

Cec was making sense! Relief washed over me, "You're back!"

"Was I gone?"

"You don't remember?"

"I opened my eyes and Mary was sitting here."

"She asked me what I was reading." Mom had tears in her eyes.

"What day is it?" Cec asked.

"Wednesday."

"What day was it before?"

"Tuesday. Do you remember the doctor who wanted to give you sleeping pills?" I asked.

"I didn't want them."

"That was yesterday."

"I went away?"

"You did."

"For how long?"

"Uh…" I did the calculation. "About eighteen hours. You don't remember?"

She shook her head.

"The sleeping pills knocked you out for a while. When you woke up you were in a delirium. You pulled out your IV." I lifted her right hand to show her the welt. "And you yanked out your stomach tube. You tried to escape. They had to restrain you."

"I don't remember."

"Any of it?"

"No."

"Good." I was relieved. She didn't remember being tied to the bed, or that I hadn't been there. "How's your pain?"

"It's there. And your mom said that Sheila is coming?"

"The doctors told me to call your family. You scared the shit out of us."

"I was that close?"

"You were that close."

I close her bank accounts and cancel her credit cards. I have the electric, gas and phone bills put in my name. I sort the papers on her desk, work documents in one pile and personal in another. I go through the drawers in her filing cabinet. In the bottom drawer are all the envelopes from the CRA, unopened.

I hadn't asked Cec what was in the envelopes from the CRA, hadn't forced an answer when she was still alive, when I still could. *Why didn't I ask? What was it that I didn't want to know?*

I pull all the letters out of the drawer and pile them on her desk. I stack them neatly into rows of five and count them.

Fifty-two.

Fifty-two unopened envelopes from the Canada Revenue Agency addressed to Cecile Georgina Kaysoe.

I count the ones sent via registered mail.

Forty-five.

I contemplate the kind of restraint, or maybe the stubbornness, that it would require to receive fifty-two registered letters from the CRA and not open a single one.

Then again, what does it take to sign for fifty-two registered letters and hand them all over without ever insisting on knowing what is in them?

Had I been honourable? Or was it denial?

I pull the letters out of the envelopes one by one: black typeface on blue paper. I sort the letters by date, from oldest to newest. I try not to read the text but I can't help seeing the word *garnishee*.

And this number: $25,838.28.

The CRA had demanded payment of $25,838.28 in back taxes because her company had done something wrong in the way they had allocated expenses. I couldn't find anything in the letters to suggest that Cec had tried to negotiate a resolution.

They'd garnisheed fifty percent of her take-home pay every month. She hadn't told me. Not a word. She'd kept on paying for our dinners out, weekends away, rounds of golf. She'd continued pulling out her credit card without hesitation. Not a blink, not a flinch, not a hint; not even in the hospital when we were discussing the status of her accounts, the bills I'd have to change over to my name.

I should have asked. Should have insisted. Should have opened one.

What had Cec called me? Naive. Too trusting. And maybe I was. I should have been more cynical. Less willing to accept her assertions at face value. I knew that Cec had no qualms about taking creative license. I'd watched her tell an outright lie with a straight face. Later she'd say, "Easier that way" or "Didn't want to get into it."

Was I foolish to have trusted?

In a box under her desk I find folders filled with her writing—stories about the farm, and travel adventures. I recognize the destinations, and some of the stories. A number are handwritten, mostly short pieces, written in the self-conscious voice of performance, as though she expected an audience.

One is about a trek across the Kalahari Desert—the first piece she ever showed me. I never questioned whether Cec actually experienced what she described. But now, for a fleeting moment, as I sit with the Kalahari story in one hand and letters from the CRA in a pile on the desk in front of me, I can't help but wonder.

On a safari in the Kalahari Desert. Myself, a guide, and two bearers. A desert like no other. No oases, no palm trees. Just rock as far as the eye can see.

We made camp before sunset. As the sun sank, the sky thickened and boiled, then flashed and cracked open wide with a flare that lit the heavens. Rain, torrential but pacific, poured down.

Rain falls on the Kalahari once every fifty years.

Just before dawn the rain stopped and the clouds disappeared. The sun arrived and I thought I had gone mad. No longer was there a barren wasteland but flowers of every shade and description, passionate and vibrant tones. Seeds and pods dormant for decades springing to life like a movie on fast-forward. Within hours the sun would destroy those fragile tendrils. That didn't matter to me.

I only needed to see it once.

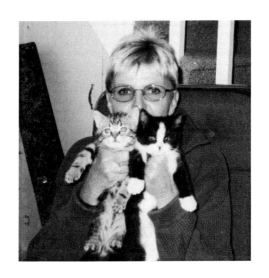

"This desire had always existed"

I lay facing the wall listening to Cec talk to the lab tech—
which arm it would be this morning—and voices mumbling
past in the hallway. The lab tech left. I heard Cec shuffling
her covers. I rolled over and squinted, rubbed sleep out of
my eye.

Jessie came into the room, followed closely by a dark-haired,
incredibly good-looking young male. "I thought I'd bring Curtis
by to introduce him," she said.

I lifted myself up onto one elbow and glanced at Cec.
She was sitting up, feet dangling over the edge of the bed,
trying to suppress a smile.

"Curtis is a student nurse. He'll be taking care of you
today," Jessie said to Cec. "I'll be supervising. I hope that's
all right with you."

"Yes," Cec said in a weakened version of her executive
voice, "that will be fine. Welcome aboard, Curtis."

"We'll be back in a bit."

"Okay."

Jessie ushered Curtis out the door and Cec grinned at
me. "If someone had told me he was being prescribed, I'd
have done my hair." She tossed her head and ran her fingers
through imaginary flowing locks.

I smiled at her obvious pleasure. Her flirtations didn't
bother me. I had no problem understanding that she could
be attracted to men, enjoy attention from them, and still be
solidly and solely with me.

I'd asked her once what it was like to sleep with a man.

"It's different."

"How is it different?"

"It just is."

I knew there was some part of her that could sleep with a man again in a heartbeat. I also knew, with certainty, that the place reserved for me at her emotional core was unalterably secure. Even so, she didn't want to admit, not to everyone, who I was in her life. In conversation with strangers, and sometimes even with friends, Cec would deliberately mention her ex-husband. I'd seen eyebrows raise and questioning glances in my direction.

Then there was the day I came home from work to find Cec in the living room holding an armload of dirty laundry. I knew before she said a word that she was feeling closed in again, furious at the clutter, even though she was the one who'd brought home virtually every ceramic bowl, candlestick, picture frame, and cookbook.

She yanked my coveralls off the back of a chair. I followed her into the bedroom.

She held up my flannel chore shirt and said, "I might as well be married to a man!"

"No!" I took my chore shirt from her. "No. You can say almost anything to me, but you cannot say *that*. If you want to be married to a man, then you go ahead. You go! Marry a man!"

"If we ever split," she said, "I'll never be with a woman again."

"Fine!"

I stomped out of the house, slammed the door, and headed to the corrals and the comfort of the animals.

When Curtis reappeared, Jessie was right behind him. "I'm here to make sure he doesn't kill you."

"They only let me do the easy jobs anyway." Curtis put his stethoscope to his ears. "Sorry, this might be a bit cold."

He listened to her heart and lungs, took her blood pressure. Jessie perched on the arm of a chair. "If you're okay with it, I'll let him come on his own next time."

"I'm sure he'll do just fine." Cec slipped off her hospital gown without hesitation so that Curtis could change the dressing under her arm. She didn't care who saw her naked. In Denmark, where all the beaches are nude beaches and the Danes much more relaxed about the naked body, Cec had done her yardwork in the buff whenever the weather permitted.

"Your shirt looks like it's from Hawaii," Cec said as Curtis taped new gauze in place. His shirt was a deep red and covered in large white flowers.

"It's not," Curtis said, "but I'd love to go. Have you been?" He finished applying the dressing and Cec pulled her gown back up

"Several times," Cec said, "but I like the beaches at Bali better, or Phuket."

"You've travelled a lot?"

I wondered for a moment whether she would begin to recount for him the many countries she'd visited. At the height of her career she'd said she was on the road more than two hundred days a year.

"I've been a few places." She was enjoying his attention, and the opportunity to have a relaxed conversation. This was what she wanted: to be treated like a normal person. I made a mental note. I would try to be less jumpy.

"Does this hurt?" He pressed against the butterfly embedded into Cec's shoulder blade.

"Not at all. You have a gentle touch."

"And you have very soft skin."

"You think so?"

"I do."

"Well, isn't that sweet of you." She batted her eyelashes.

"Not at all." He gave a little bow. "Ready for your morphine?"

"Yes, please."

"I'll be right back."

As soon as he left the room, Cec said, with mock affectation, "I have very soft skin."

"Yes, you do, Babe." I couldn't help smiling.

"Yes, I most certainly do. Could you bring me my hairbrush?"

I got her brush from the bathroom. Then I pulled her purse out of the locker, found her red lipstick, and held it up. "Would you like this too?"

She shook her head, grinning. "Don't want to scare the poor boy."

Curtis returned with a syringe. Cec leaned forward so he could insert the needle into her butterfly.

"You do that like a pro," Cec said.

"My mother taught me."

"She was a nurse?"

"No. She, uh, she had breast cancer. I took care of her. I wasn't a nurse then, but it's where I learned—"

"Oh, I—"

"It's okay. That was a few years ago. She passed away."

"I'm sorry."

"How's that? Can you feel it?"

Cec closed her eyes and took a deep breath, "There it is. Thank you."

My cellphone began to vibrate. I stepped out of Cec's room. I wouldn't take my cell out of my pocket or check who it was until I was out of earshot. I answered in a hushed voice as I walked down the pale blue hall past the nurses' station and out into the main flesh-coloured corridor. It was Doreen.

"I have bad news," she said.

The farm.

"Two big black dogs came onto the yard. They got into the chicken run."

"What black dogs?"

"I don't know where they came from but they were huge."

"How many did they get?"

"Almost all of them."

Griff had managed to get into one of the chicken runs once. We'd stacked some bales too close and he'd jumped up onto the stack and over the fence into the run. He'd killed all the chickens. Every single one.

When I got home from work that day, Griff was still inside the run whining to get out. It had taken me a minute to realize that the feathery lumps on the ground were dead chickens. I shrieked at him. When I opened the gate, I tackled him to the ground, grabbed the loose fur around his neck and shook him. But it didn't matter. It was too late.

"Both runs?"

"And one of the goats."

"A goat?!"

"They killed her."

"Which one?"

"The black one with the white on her chin."

"Tremble. She was one of Cec's favorites." A bossy little nanny.

"When we drove onto the yard one of the dogs came running to meet us. The other one was working on the goat. She was already dead. I don't think they're strays. They're too friendly."

"Any idea who they belong to?"

"No. Hank called Jake. He came with his gun. One of the dogs took off. Jake got the other one."

"I'm glad Griff and Charlie weren't there."

"Griff would have tried to protect the farm. He wouldn't have stood a chance."

"Do you think the other one will come back?"

"I don't know. Jake said that he'll keep checking your place. Can't have dogs killing livestock."

I didn't even have to ask. Doreen would load the chickens and Tremble into the back of her pickup. She had come on the day of the Griff massacre and we'd done that grim job together.

Cec's eyes were closed, the lights dimmed. I changed into pajama bottoms, pulled off my fleecy. I undid my bra, put on a T-shirt.

I hadn't told Cec about the black dogs, or the dead chickens, or Tremble. I wouldn't. I wanted her to remember the farm intact.

I went into Cec's little bathroom and examined my face in the mirror. Dark shadows had gathered under my eyes. I moved my toothbrush up and down over my teeth. My mouth filled with peppermint froth. I rinsed and spat, took another long look. My cheeks were sunken and pale. Was it the fluorescent lighting that made me look gaunt?

Everything in my expression—eyes, cheeks, lips— turned downwards. I hadn't noticed before. My eyes looked sad. This was what Cec saw when she looked at me. No wonder it was easier for her when I wasn't around.

I wandered out into the hallway. It was a small comfort to walk away from the gurgle of the oxygen pump, the muted beep of the IV monitor.

I stopped at the nurses' station to confirm the time for Cec's next round then went out of the ward into the main hallway to call Mom. The last time we'd talked she'd said that Cher, my sister, might come.

I watched an older woman, hunched and bowed, pushing a man in a wheelchair. His eyes were closed, head bobbing.

They must think I'm a patient too, I thought, as I stood there in my pajamas, hair askew. Did they wonder about my illness? How long I'd been in here? Whether my case was terminal?

I faced the wall, curled into a fetal ball, pulled the blankets up around my face. My cot was too short, the mattress hard and thin. The wire mesh pressed into my arm. I couldn't let myself surrender to sleep. Cec might need a nurse. Or she might want to move from the recliner to the bed. Or she might have to go to the bathroom.

I commanded myself to stop thinking. Fragmented images floated. The feathers of dead chickens. Black dogs chasing the goats in their small pen. The goats scattering, and bleeting, terrified.

I closed my eyes, to shut out the thought of Tremble, and saw the dead baby moose. She had tried to follow her mother over a barbed-wire fence. One of her back legs got caught and she went down, her leg tangled in the wire. She'd flailed under a hot sun until she'd worn the grass down to dirt. By the time we found her, she was stiff.

The hardest of all was Annie.

"You'll have to keep an eye on her," Cec said as she packed for a business trip. Annie's udder was red, but no sores. "Make sure you manually express milk out of every quadrant, a couple times a day." I'd nodded but I wasn't optimistic. Annie didn't appreciate human hands on her teats. She barely tolerated her own calf.

Because there were no sores, I thought maybe she just had a mild case of mastitis or a bit of a rash. I was half-hearted in my attempts to milk her.

Annie grew listless. Then she stopped eating. No interest in oats? I called Andy, the vet. He said that it could be mastitis even without the sores. By the time he arrived, Annie's breathing was laboured. The infection had moved into her bloodstream.

Andy gave her antibiotics and said we'd have to cross our fingers that she had it in her to fight off the infection.

I called Cec. She caught the next flight, a day early. By the time Cec got home, Annie was on her side, panting hard, tongue hanging out the side of her mouth, eyes rolled up into her head.

Cec called Andy, then sent me into town to get feed and supplies from the lumberyard. We both knew what was coming. Cec didn't want me there.

When I drove back onto the yard a couple of hours later, I saw Andy come out of the small corral wearing long plastic gloves and a plastic yellow apron. His gloves and apron both had blood on them. Cec followed him out of the corral.

"We had to put her down," Cec said to me when I walked up to them. "She didn't go easy."

"It's surprising sometimes how hard it can be," Andy said. "But we had no choice. She was too far gone."

Friday, March 11

Dr. Steader assumed a stiff stance. "I've consulted with the palliative team and they agree that a thoracentesis would relieve the pressure on her lungs."

"A thora—what?"

He stood tapping his pen on the metal railing of Cec's bed. Where had he learned his bedside manners?

"Please don't," I said to him, pointing at his pen. He stuck it back in his lab coat.

"A thoracentesis is a way to drain fluid from around the lungs. Ascites are—"

"Ascites?"

"That's the fluid building up around her lungs—"

I indicated that he should talk to Cec.

"Or, I mean," he turned to Cec, "your lungs."

"What would it involve?" she asked.

"I'd insert a needle between your ribs and suck out the fluid."

"Will it hurt?" I asked.

"No. I'd give her, I mean you," he said to Cec, "a local anaesthetic. You'd feel a bit of pressure."

"What are the risks?"

"The very worst case would be a punctured lung. But you don't need to worry, I've done this procedure many times before. The risk is minimal."

"What do you think?" Cec asked, looking at me.

"You know how much your breathing is compromised. If he thinks this will help…"

"Where would you do it?" Cec turned back to Steader.

"Right here, in your room." I could see he was getting fidgety. He wanted her to agree so he could get on with it.

Cec's mind was churning, slowly.

"I'd want you to stay with me," Cec said to me. Then to Steader, "I'd want her here."

"Not a problem."

"When?"

"Later this morning. As soon as I can set it up."

I could just imagine Dr. Daniel Steader showing up at Cec's office for a job interview. She'd size him up—his strut, his biceps, his stiff words—and she'd cut the interview short. No way she'd hire him. But here he was, full of his own importance and in charge of her care.

Steader had Cec sit on the edge of her bed and lean forward, rest her elbows on the bedside table. A tall, balding young intern, who had come in with Steader, was decked out in full surgery attire, including a hairnet and face mask. The hairnet seemed like overkill.

I sat facing Cec on a rolling stool that I'd found in the hallway. The stool was high enough that I could rest my arms on her bedside table and hold her hands.

Cec squeezed her eyes shut and clenched her jaw when the needle went in.

"Does it hurt?"

"No."

I closed my eyes, trying to banish the thought of that long needle from my mind, and think about something happy, pleasant: Cec in her hot-pink dress and burgundy pumps.

"You okay?" Cec squeezed my hand.

"I'm okay."

"What are you thinking about?"

"Nothing. Just trying to relax."

"You're a bit tense."

"We're almost there," Steader said.

He held up a litre of pale yellow liquid. It looked a lot like pee.

"Take a deep breath," he said to Cec.

She sat up straight and inhaled a long, slow breath. "Yes, that's better."

The day I moved in with Cec she insisted on making a special dinner in celebration. She refused my help, shooed me out of the kitchen.

I sat in the living room waiting for her to call me for dinner, feeling like a guy. The aroma of gravy and stuffing wafted in my direction. She took off her apron and went into the bedroom, closed the door, emerged wearing a hot-pink dress, a pearl necklace and heels. She walked back into the kitchen without a glance in my direction and continued stirring the gravy.

I got up off the couch and stood in the kitchen doorway. "Hey!"

She turned.

"You look hot!"

Then I really felt like a guy, standing there with my hands in my pockets. I wanted, more than anything, to take her in my arms, kiss her, but I hesitated, surprised by the intensity of my desire.

I'd always known that I was attracted to the masculine in Cec—her calm certainty, her virility, her ability to handle power tools. But there I stood, attracted to the curve of her, the round of her breasts, the plunge of her hot-pink neckline. I was attracted to the feminine in her. A startling surprise. And not a surprise at all. Looking back I could see that this desire had always existed, in a demure and bashful form, waiting to be acknowledged.

Mom hugged me first. I couldn't hold back the tears. Dad had called me on my cell when they'd arrived at the hospital, and I met them as they were coming out of the elevator.

Cher opened her arms. My sister. Six years younger than me, an inch and a half taller, and the most sensitive person I know.

When we were kids, all I had to do was lift my eyes from my cereal bowl and Cher would wail, "Don't look at me like thaaat—"

"I'm not looking at you!"

"There!" Mom would set a Cheerios box between us. "Now you two don't have to look at each other."

As we both got older, and our communication became more adult, I realized that we related to the world and the people around us in a very similar way. Conversations with Cher could go on for hours. She was expressive, and engaging, and needed to hear herself speak to make sense of life.

Cher entered Cec's room first. "Oh, come here, my girl," Cec waved her over to the bed.

Cher had spent several summers in Calgary and had often come golfing with us. It was on the golf course, where the only real concern was the trajectory of a small white ball, that Cec had come to appreciate Cher's gentleness, her genuine curiosity, her ability to laugh at herself.

"It's just not right," Cher said wiping away tears and trying to smile, "you lying around in bed in the middle of the day."

"Maybe we should go," Mom said. "Give Cher and Cec some time."

"It's okay," Cher said.

"Sit, Mary." Cec motioned toward the chairs.

"No, we'll go for coffee. Okay, Richard? Would you like to come too, Lyn?"

"I just want to sleep," I said, dropping onto my cot.

Mom and Dad left and I curled up on top of rumpled blankets. The afternoon sun was high in the sky and the room was growing warm. I closed my eyes.

I don't know how long I slept. Maybe minutes. Felt like days.

Eventually I surfaced, slowly, from oblivion into warmth and murmur. I heard a faraway voice say, "I don't know how you can—"

"It is what is it, my girl." Cec's voice was hoarse.

A muffled shuffling. My eyelids were heavy, my mouth dry, shoulder sore.

"I wouldn't…I couldn't…" Cher's voice quavered.

"No point fighting…" Cec's voice trailed off.

"How come I'm mad but you're not?"

"Mad at what?"

"That you're in here. Like this."

"No. No, sshhh." Cec was shushing Cher like she shushed me. "We have an understanding."

"We?"

"Me and God. I've always been there for him."

"But he's supposed to be there for you!"

"He is. This isn't punishment."

Cher blew her nose.

"It's like…" Cec paused. "I've been playing on one team, now he's asking me to switch sides."

I opened my eyes. I could make out the blurry shape of Cher leaning against the windowsill dabbing at her eyes.

Cec reached out her hand and Cher took it. "No sense fighting it, or being mad."

I closed my eyes again and let my mind sink into the dark irrational cave of semi-consciousness. Cec's calm assurance was comforting.

I must have tipped over into sleep. When I opened my eyes again, Mom and Dad had returned. They were talking in whispers with Cher.

Sanjay entered softly, sensing a full room. Dr. Choy was with him.

Mom got up. "We should go."

"No, stay," I said, sitting up. Cec waved at her to sit down.

"There's no room."

"Pull the recliner over."

"I'll sit with you." Mom motioned for me to move my legs so she could perch on the end of my cot.

Sanjay nodded and introduced himself and Dr. Choy to my parents and sister.

"I'll be going on holiday tomorrow," Sanjay said. "Dr. Choy will be in charge of your care while I'm away."

"Could you tell them to bring me real food?" Cec asked.

"Are you hungry?" Choy asked. Sanjay had stepped back as though on cue. "That's a good sign." Choy nodded approvingly.

"Sick of Jell-O."

"Well, since you've had a few bowel movements—"

"Yes!" Cec gave a small fist pump. "Bowel movements!"

"—you can try solids again. We'll see how your system tolerates—"

"I want to go home."

"Home?"

"To the farm."

"Oh yes, your farm. Where is it?"

"An hour's drive," I said.

Choy made a note.

"I'll have to have home care," Cec said.

Choy nodded contemplatively. I sat up straighter. *Was he going to send her home?*

"I have three concerns," Choy said. He held up three fingers and touched his left index finger to his right index finger. "First is transportation. It will be difficult for you to make a long trip, especially on country roads—"

"There's pavement all the way, except the last mile." Cec had thought about this.

"Even so, travel is a challenge, especially if you are in pain. As you already know, pain can be difficult to predict, and even harder to control."

Cec didn't say anything. She knew.

"I also have a concern about your pain management." He paused as though anticipating a counter-argument. "A number of factors can contribute to rapid pain escalation."

"You could stay with us," Mom piped up.

Cec and I turned to her.

"But your guest room is downstairs, Mom."

"I can't do stairs," Cec said, "but that's a lovely offer, Mary. Thank you."

"We'd move into the guest room, wouldn't we, Richard? You could have our bedroom. The bathroom is right there."

A collective silence of hesitation. Then Cec said, "That's very generous."

"And worth considering," Choy continued. "Particularly since my third concern is distance to the nearest hospital."

Listening to Choy I let myself wonder, for the first time, what would happen if she lived on in this state, sometimes better, sometimes worse, for months? Years? I had to shut that thought out. Life outside the pale-blue walls of this hospital room already felt distant. Marion had said that Cec's world would get smaller. Mine had too.

Cec waved her hand for Choy to stop talking. "Forget it. Lyn doesn't want me at home."

"Of course I do!" I heard myself say the words and

simultaneously felt the rapid rise of terror at the thought of being alone with her in our farmhouse with the drafty windows and the uneven floors. *What if it snowed and we couldn't get out?* Or the electricity might go out like it did sometimes. I could see myself standing at the patio doors looking out at an empty expanse of prairie, snow swirling.

"You really would be welcome at our house." My mother's expression was a mix of earnest concern and eagerness to help.

"I know, Mary, and thank you, but I wouldn't want to put you out."

"We'd need to do an assessment," Choy interjected.

"Not sure I could manage your front steps," Cec said.

"There would be a number of factors." Choy was making notes. "Another option to consider may be hospice care."

I saw a flash of sadness (or maybe resignation?) in Cec's eyes.

"But not if you are undergoing treatment."

"And we don't know yet, about treatment," Cec said. "I haven't seen the oncologist." Her appointment had been rescheduled for March fourteenth.

"You would have to be prepared to agree to end-of-life care."

"What does that mean?" I asked.

"A cessation of treatment."

"Is that the same as a DNR?"

"No, a DNR is level three. It means no intervention in the case of an event."

"There it is again," Cec said with a shake of her head. "Level three."

"End-of-life care means that you would not be receiving active treatment."

"But she would still get morphine."

"Of course. We would do everything possible to keep you comfortable."

"Wouldn't it be best to wait with making a decision until Cec has seen the oncologist?"

"Level three," Cec said.

Choy and I looked at her.

"Three," she said again. "No to 'end-of-life care,' not yet, but yes to 'three.' I'll sign."

"Are you sure? You don't have to—"

"It makes the most sense."

"I'll have a nurse bring the paperwork."

"Paperwork. Of course. Even for the dying."

Saturday, March 12

In typical Cecile fashion, all she had told Franz (her VP of sales and the person she reported to) was that she had to have minor surgery and would be away for a few days. I had said to her, several times, in her moments of coherency, that I thought she should provide a few more details, "so that the seriousness of your situation won't come as such a surprise."

"Why? We don't really know yet. And besides, this is personal."

I'm not sure what finally convinced her. Maybe the delerium—realizing how close she'd come.

I watched her click rapidly on the computer keys.

"Here." She glanced up. "You get your wish. Read this before I hit SEND."

From: Cecile Kaysoe
Sent: Saturday, March 12, 2005 12:11 PM
To: Franz Allek
Subject: Situation

Hi Franz,

My sincere apologies for not being quicker at updating you but events have been moving ahead very rapidly.

In the course of the recent surgery it was discovered that I have cancer. I have been waiting for the pathology and am still in hospital. The pathologies have come back now, and I apparently have a very serious and aggressive Stage Four cancer. At the same time I also picked up a couple of infections that have complicated the situation. I have been right out of it for many days—today being the first time that I have been able to respond—even on a limited basis. My family has been called in from various points around the world, and we will have an opportunity to discuss things in the course of this weekend.

As you can imagine—I am in a state of shock, and don't really know what I am doing right now. My cell is on now, as well as my email.

I have no idea time lines or any other details at this stage. We have a consultation with the cancer clinic here next week to figure out the way forward. Any advice you can give me as to what I do now would be great.

Rgds,
Cecile

"Good." I handed the laptop back to her. "It's better he knows. Are you cold?"

Cec was sitting on the edge of the bed. Her feet looked blue.

"I have to do this while I have the minutes." She was hunched over her laptop, a blonde elf in a hospital gown. A few more clicks and the email was sent.

"Here, take this," she passed me her laptop, "and help me…" I lifted her swollen legs onto the bed, one at at time, then arranged her blankets.

"Come here." Cec motioned for me to come closer. "Sit with me."

I pulled a chair as close as I could. She reached for my hand then closed her eyes. I sat with her cool, limp hand in mine studying her face. When I closed my eyes, her face would dissolve. I couldn't bring it back. I opened my eyes again and tried to imprint her face on my memory.

I was about to lay her hand on the bed when she squeezed. "You still here?"

"Should I go? Do you want to sleep?"

"Stay."

She looked so relaxed. Maybe this was a good time to ask. "What do you think is on the other side?"

She opened her eyes. "The other side?"

"Do you think there is life after—"

"You've written me off?"

"No. It's just—"

"We're not there yet." She let go of my hand.

We weren't? What about level three? And Plan B?

Cec had been standing at the patio door one afternoon watching a torrential downpour when I heard her say, "Thanks, Mom." She turned to me. "I told her we needed rain."

"Your mother sent this?"

"She's still mad about being dead. She likes having something to do."

I should have asked Cec where she thought her mother was. Floating about in some kind of hereafter? Not heaven in the classic Christian sense. Not for Cec. Or me. I couldn't imagine that.

"You don't have to worry, Lyn." Cec was reaching for my hand again. "I'll always be with you, you know that."

My throat tightened. I let her take my hand and hoped she couldn't see the panic in my eyes.

Would she be able to read my mind? Know everything? What I was really thinking? And feeling?

The thought terrified me. Even though she'd always had a strong intuition, a sixth sense about what I wasn't willing to admit. She understood my motivations, my manipulations. She knew the ways in which I was pretending. And this hurt her.

It was in part my guilt that had kept me rooted, trying to prove myself. I suspected that if I did ever manage to prove to Cec that I loved her in the way she wanted me to, it might make it harder to leave. But as long as we were together, I needed to try.

I met Marion in the hallway and stood talking with her at the nursing station, anxious to get back to Cec but also needing, for the space of a few deep breaths, the comfort of her solid presence.

"How are you?" I had the sense, as I usually did when I saw Marion, that she wanted to put her hand on my arm. She could see I was coming unhinged, and that human touch was one of the few ways to steady to me. But I think she could also tell that I was raw and couldn't tolerate much contact. When I would walk down the hall with my eyes down, one of the nurses would sometimes come toward me. I'd wave her away, "Please, no," afraid that I would come completely undone if she put her arm around me. As long as Cec was still hanging on, I needed to hang on too.

"Her pain is...vicious. I don't know how much longer I can do this."

"I think you're stronger than you know."

"You've seen a lot of people die?"

She nodded. "I've lived my career in the grey zone between life and death."

"Are many in pain? At the end?"

"Some, yes. Others slip away quietly."

"But not with cancer."

"Even with cancer. Some types of cancer aren't painful."

"But—I thought—" I hadn't expected this. "I thought cancer was always painful."

"Sometimes there's no pain at all." Her eyes squinted as though she was trying to see whether I was ready to hear what she was going to say next. "When someone is in extreme pain at the end, it's often more psychological than physical."

"What do you mean, psychological?"

"I'm not saying that the pain isn't physical. I know it is. But when pain is extreme there's often a deeper reason, something that needs to be resolved."

A deeper reason? Cec seemed so accepting, matter-of-fact. She didn't seem unresolved.

But I knew there was much I didn't know. All I had to go on were the pieces she'd told me, her version of those stories.

If I'd known what to ask, if she had been willing to talk, what would she have said? Was there some personal devastation she'd kept buried? Something she'd done that she regretted? I'd never know. All I knew was that she was reaching for my hand more often. I felt her vulnerability in her weakened grip and it created a pull, like a gravitational force. That pull had always been there but it was stronger now, and permeated with a sense of foreboding.

I hadn't walked away when I could have. And now there was only one exit.

"I'm afraid that I'll be there when she…" I took a deep breath. "And then I'm afraid that…I won't."

Marion didn't say anything. Her silence was comforting.

"How many people have you seen die?" I asked.

She didn't answer right away. "Maybe…a hundred?"

"You were with all of them? Right at the end?"

"I was."

I wanted to ask what that was like, but I didn't. She couldn't tell me what I really wanted to know anyway: how it would be for me.

"I'm not very good at this."

"Most people…" Marion lowered her voice. "Even when

you know it's coming, you can never really be prepared for the permanence."

Permanence.

I realized then that I had been expecting—not consciously, but in the way that the body anticipates—that there would always be a wide steel hospital door and Cec's skinny-bloated body in a half-raised bed.

"I make Cec tense. She doesn't want me around."

"She's probably anxious."

"She's incredibly calm, actually."

"She's very fortunate to have you."

"I don't think she…" I shook my head.

"She is. Even if she can't say it."

I reached her room at the end of the hall. I stopped and took a deep breath before I pushed open her door. The window was letting in so much light that Cec seemed to be glowing, her hair a bright, translucent white.

I wanted to crawl into bed beside her. The desire was overwhelming. I wanted to open my arms to the weight of her head against my chest, breathe in her hot-sour breath. I wanted to fall asleep to the syncopated rise and fall of our breathing, her thin body stretched out alongside mine, fading but still warm.

Sunday, March 13

I was sitting cross-legged on my cot, leaning back against the cool of cement brick wall. Sheila, Cec's sister from Long Island, was telling Cec about a meditation retreat she'd been to.

I heard Cec say, "I'm so fortunate."

Fortunate?

"I say that I want Lyn here with me, and she's here." Cec was smiling. "How many people have that?"

I waited. For the bite of sarcasm.

"She's a good nurse," Cec said.

A good nurse? Was she talking about me?

"She gets my ice, and hot water for tea, even though I almost never drink it."

I looked at Sheila. She was giving me the kind of smile generally reserved for small children who have just performed in a Christmas pageant.

Was I supposed to say something?

I didn't have the energy, not now when we were hurtling toward—I saw Sanjay's fingers floating along, then pointing downward. She could have offered this up sooner, when her gratitude could have made us stronger.

What was I supposed to do with this now?

I was edgy, and irritated. Mad that she was dying. Furious at her gratitude. Guilty that I was mad.

Cec couldn't get comfortable, even with an increase in morphine. Her pain didn't seem to be snowballing but it wasn't settling either.

She opened her eyes and sat up, flapping her hands. "Get her off!"

"Who?" I stood up and moved closer.

"She's tickling my legs."

"Who is?"

"The kitten. You need to take her."

I moved to the other side of Cec's bed. "Cec, it's Lyn. You're in the hospital. The kittens are at the farm."

Cec glared at me and kicked her leg. "You're not helping!"

"I think you're having a dream."

"She's rubbing me." Cec patted at her chest. "Ohhh, she's so cute…" Her eyes closed again and her head fell to the side.

The next time Cec opened her eyes she said, "I just wanted one more."

"Morphine?"

"One more round of golf."

I moved closer to the bed and took her hand.

"I birdied the last hole," she said.

"You did?"

"At Valley Ridge. The last time we played. Remember?"

The last round of golf we had played had been at Valley Ridge. She wasn't hallucinating.

"I hit a beautiful drive."

I couldn't remember her drive.

"You don't remember."

"I don't."

"My second shot landed on the green."

I didn't remember that either.

"One putt," Cec said. "It was a par 4. We were playing with your dad."

I remembered my father hitting some wild shots on the

last couple of holes. His tee shots could go wayward when he got tired.

"You don't remember my birdie?"

I shook my head. I didn't. I wished I did.

"You were too busy being frustrated with yourself."

I probably was.

Monday, March 14

Dr. Steader arrived before the sun was up, before the lab tech. He entered the room with a bounce in his step.

"I've scheduled you for an MRI," he said cheerfully. "Your appointment with the oncologist will have to be rescheduled."

"Again?" *Just like that?*

Cec flashed me a grin. She had been trying to convince someone that she needed an MRI since the pain first started.

"If the MRI shows bone cancer then we might be able to treat it with radiation and this might alleviate some of your pain," he said to Cec, who was nodding.

"What about the appointment with the oncologist?" I stood.

"If they can figure out my pain…" Cec gripped my arm, urging me to sit.

"Your MRI is scheduled for noon but if they have an opening sooner, they'll come and get you." Steader was obviously pleased with himself.

"Can't they do the MRI another day? Tomorrow?"

"Her appointment at the cancer centre has already been cancelled."

"What about morphine?" Cec asked.

She and I both knew: one shot would not be enough. And she was going to have to lie flat for an MRI. Had she thought about that? The thought made me queasy.

Steader assured her that she'd get her shot. They'd give

her the maximum just before she went down. He'd order extra morphine tablets to send with her, just in case.

"A porter will come for you when they're ready so you won't have to wait."

"How long will it take?"

"About thirty minutes."

"Thirty minutes?!"

Cec couldn't even lie flat for thirty seconds. How in the world did anyone think she would make it through thirty minutes?

"It'll be okay," Cec said, waving at me. "Don't get yourself all worked up."

"When will she go to the cancer centre?"

"I'll let you know as soon as a new appointment has been confirmed."

Jessie stuck her head in the door. "A porter is on his way. To take you down for your MRI."

"Where's Curtis?"

"What?! I'm not good enough for you anymore? I'll be right back with your shot. Don't let them take you before you get that. And your pills."

My heartrate accelerated. This was it. They were coming.

Jessie delivered a top-up injection of morphine and gave Cec two small white morphine tablets in a little plastic container to take with her. *Only two?* That wouldn't be enough.

The porter arrived pushing a gurney. He wanted Cec to lie on it.

"She can't lie flat!" I stepped between the porter and Cec. "Can't you take her in a wheelchair?"

Cec was nodding. "That would be better. Or I could sit on that."

"No, a gurney isn't made for someone to sit on. You'll have to lie down."

"I'll push her in a wheelchair."

"Wheelchairs aren't supposed to leave the ward." The porter was getting impatient.

"I'll bring it back."

"But it—"

"I'll get permission."

The porter pursed his lips. I could see that it went against everything in him to break the rules.

I pulled Cec's slippers onto her feet and helped her pull on a housecoat. I got a wheelchair from the hallway and helped her into it.

"You have the pills?"

She lifted her clenched fist. "Go!"

The porter took the lead, pushing the empty gurney down to the basement and into IMAGING. He rolled the gurney into a curtained stall and indicated that we should wait there. The porter walked down a short hallway and stuck his head in a doorway. When he came back he said, "Someone will be with you shortly. You'll need to get onto that." He was pointing at the gurney.

"She will when she has to," I said. The porter was deeply reluctant to leave her sitting in the wheelchair but he turned, finally, and walked away.

A nurse or a lab technician, a woman, appeared with a clipboard.

"You'll need to lie on the bed," she said.

"It's very painful for her to lie down. Better if she waits until right before she goes in."

"You'll need to lie on your back for about thirty minutes," the woman said to Cec. "Will you be able to do that?"

Cec nodded.

"Is there anyway to do the MRI in less than thirty minutes?" I asked.

"Not for the number of images requested."

"How long before she goes in?"

"About fifteen minutes. I'll need you to fill this out." She handed Cec the clipboard. "If you are wearing earrings or a watch, anything metal, it's very important that you take them off. Do you have any metal implants? Pins? Pacemaker?"

Cec shook her head, no. Her face was flushed.

"We were told that she wouldn't have to wait, that she'd be brought down and would go right in."

"It shouldn't be too much longer," the woman said. "Fill that out and I'll be right back."

I took the clipboard from Cec and read through the checklist of medical conditions. Stage four ovarian cancer wasn't on the list. I filled out the form and gave it to Cec to sign. She waved it away, "You sign."

"Me?"

"It doesn't matter."

I signed. Where was the nurse? "You need your pills?"

"I need a shot." The colour had drained from her face.

"You want the pills or should I take you back up?"

"The pills." She had her arms around her middle and was rocking back and forth.

"I'll find water."

I went to where that the porter had reported in. Two young women were sitting in front of a row of computer screens, their backs to me. They were looking through a large window at the MRI machine that was making a whirring sound. Cec would have to wait until this person was finished.

"I'm with a patient who's in a lot of pain and waiting for an MRI. How long will it be?"

The women turned. One of them looked back at the computer screens. The other one said, "About fifteen minutes."

"Fifteen minutes?! I can tell you right now she won't last that long. We were told she'd be taken right in."

"I don't know who said that."

I could tell her who! "Is there somewhere I can get a glass of water?"

"Down the hall. There's a fountain."

I'd seen paper cups in the stall where Cec's gurney stood waiting. I grabbed one and got some water. Cec swallowed the pills.

"I don't know if they'll stay down," she said. I looked around for a basin.

"How much longer?"

"They said about ten minutes."

Cec sucked in a short, sharp breath. As she exhaled, she said, "Stop fidgeting!"

"They said they'd take you right in." I shifted from one foot to the other.

"Well, they're liars. And you're not helping. Relax! Or go away."

I thought about going to get Jessie. But that would take too long. I tried to stand still, my back to Cec. I heard her mumble.

"What, Babe?"

"I can't. I just can't."

"You want to go back up?"

She nodded.

"I'll tell them."

The young women looked surprised when I said I was taking Cec back to the ward. I didn't wait to hear what they had to say.

I rolled Cec into her room and helped her from the wheelchair to the pink recliner. Her face was pale, her breathing laboured. I went to find Curtis. He was with Jessie, tending a patient. Jessie told him to carry on and went to get the morphine.

"Jessie is on her way," I said to Cec, breathless. She was gripping the armrest of the recliner, her eyes closed.

She said, "You need to go—buy me pajamas."

"Now?"

"Bottoms. XL"

"But—"

"Go!" She opened her eyes, glared at me. "You're too jumpy."

"But—"

"When Jessie comes."

And then Jessie was in the room.

"Keep an eye on her," I said.

"You okay?" Jessie reached for me but I was heading for the door.

"I have to go."

"She's fine," Cec said to Jessie. "You have my drugs?"

When I got back to Cec's room, her bed was empty. Lora was standing beside Cec's empty bed, her back to the door. When she turned, I could see she'd been crying.

"It's not fair," she said.

"No, it's not. Where is she?"

"One of the doctor's came. They sent her for an MRI."

"Did someone go with her?"

"The doctor did. Said he wanted to make sure she had enough morphine."

"I think I need a smoke," I said, shoving my hands into my pockets.

"Are you serious?" Lora looked at me with surprise.

"No, I'm not serious. But if I were going to become a smoker, this would be a good time to start. I could seriously use a bad habit right now."

"Cec said she was ten or eleven when she started to chauffeur your father," I said quietly. I was sitting in the visitors' room with Sheila, Cec's sister from Long Island.

"She wasn't that young. More like fourteen."

"She said she could barely reach the pedals."

"I'm pretty sure she had her learner's."

"Really?" This wasn't adding up. Cec said that she'd moved out at fourteen.

"Cec said she'd drive your dad to the Cecil Hotel and wait for him in the truck until three or four in the morning."

"Did she? Yeah, that could have happened."

"But you don't remember how old she was—"

"I remember her buying a car. I got home from school one day and she and my dad had their heads under the hood. It was blue, I think."

"On her sixteenth birthday?"

"Was that her birthday?"

"Your mom said that Cec skipped school on her sixteenth birthday, got her licence, bought a car, and got car insurance. Then she drove the car home and said to your dad, 'So, what'd you think?'"

Sheila shook her head. "I don't remember it being her birthday."

"But you remember the car."

"Vaguely. I think it was hers."

"What about when she was little and she wanted to wear her holster and guns to a birthday party? Or maybe you were too young."

Sheila's brow furrowed.

"Cec said she was about five or six. Your mom sent her upstairs to put on a dress to go to a birthday party. She came down in the dress with her holster and guns strapped around her waist. Your mom told her to take off the holster."

"I don't remember. Was my dad there?"

"Cec said he laughed and said there wasn't any harm in a couple of toy guns."

"What I remember," Sheila said, "is Cec showing up one day, she was maybe nine, with a case of beer under her arm."

I could imagine a nine-year-old Cec lugging a case of beer. And I couldn't. Had this really happened or was this a family fable?

"How does a nine-year-old get a hold of a case of beer?"

"No idea. That was Cec, infinitely resourceful."

"What did your parents say?"

"They were both drinking pretty heavily by then. I don't think either of them really noticed."

"What did Cec say?"

"Nothing. She just put the beer on the kitchen table and went out to play."

Sanjay brought the MRI results almost immediately: "Good news! No cancer in your bones." His tone was triumphant.

I couldn't look at him. *I knew that MRI would be pointless!*

There was scant relief on Cec's face. The absence of cancer in her bones left her without an explanation for the pain in her back.

I think Sanjay had expected a more enthusiastic response.

I needed to pace, but I couldn't. Not yet. Not while Sanjay was still here. I was mad that Cec had let Steader move her appointment.

I felt like throwing up. If there was a way to expel this— this venom—from my stomach, from my mind... I sank down onto my cot and put my head between my knees, furious with myself. I was incompetent at being mad, abysmal at anger. I'd never learned how.

My pacifist parents didn't fight. They preferred to tiptoe around what they really wanted to say. As a child I had sat at many a tense dinner table swallowing malignant particles of unarticulated rage with my mashed potatoes.

My dad would eat quickly, leave the table, disappear behind his newspaper and fall asleep on the couch. Later, at some unrelated and unanticipated moment, he'd explode about a set of waylaid keys or a bike left on the lawn.

My mother preferred the art of the ambush. When Dad got home from work she'd say, "Notice anything different, dear?"

I'd stop whatever I was doing and pretend not to watch.

He'd get that Oh shit! deer-in-headlights look, "Uh, the house looks great—?"

Wrong! She had weeded the garden. Or cleaned the garage.

I swallowed hard, and swallowed again, my rage coagulating into guilt. Guilt that I'd thought about leaving. Guilt that I wished I'd left. Guilt that I wasn't dying.

How sick was she? How long could she hang on? Would they send her home?

I squeezed my eyes tight. I hadn't left. I was glad I hadn't, so I could be here. But still—I hadn't told her what I was really thinking, so many times. I had hovered on the periphery, maintained a rationalized barrier of protection, never stepped fully in, never completely engaged. Cec had sensed this and it had hurt her.

Somewhere in the back of my mind I held an understanding that her irritation with me, her constant dissatisfaction, was this unspoken knowing—that I'd stayed in my head, that my relationship with her had been a calculation. I found her fascinating, intriguing. I loved her. But I'd never been truly, madly, head-over-heels.

"The MRI was useless! I knew it would be."

"Wasn't useless," Cec lifted her head from the pillow.

Dr. Choy was consulting a paper covered in fine, precise handwriting. "Your appointment with the gyne-oncologist has been re-scheduled for Thursday, the seventeenth."

"The seventeenth?!"

"That's in two days," he said gently.

"It's the second time her appointment has been moved. And for what!?"

"We know there's no cancer in her bones."

"Relax, Lyn. You're too jumpy." Cec put her hand on my arm. I jerked my arm away. I couldn't let myself relax. If I relaxed, I'd cry. If I started to cry, I wasn't sure I would be able to stop.

Choy said, "It is my opinion that your pain has not been well-controlled. In part that is because you want to keep your morphine low."

"Don't like the dreams," Cec mumbled.

"We could better manage the hallucinations if we changed you over to Fentanyl."

Cec shook her head, just barely.

"She had an allergic reaction last time!"

Why did they keep insisting when they knew that Cec wouldn't agree? Wasn't there a different drug they could give her?

"We don't know that for sure."

"No Fentanyl!" Cec lifted her head from the pillow, her voice stronger than I'd heard in many days.

"Okay. Then we need to look at other variables. Your constipation. We need to see whether we can get your bowels functioning."

"I had a poop."

"But you're still not regular. And the morphine will continue to slow your system. I know that laxatives haven't worked well, or the enemas. This isn't surprising given the advanced status of your cancer and the length of time you've been on morphine. If you are willing, I have a suggestion for another approach." Cec didn't respond so Choy looked at me. "I think we should try Octreotide. It's a steroid. It will help to stimulate bowel function."

The hum of the HVAC was working on me like a cocoon. I wanted to sleep, suddenly, compulsively.

I motioned toward Cec. He should ask her.

"If you are willing," he said to Cec, "I'll start you on Octreotide. I have great confidence it will help. And regardless of the effectiveness, the steroid will not create pressure the way that the enema did."

Cec opened her eyes. "I don't take steroids."

"This is a very specific application. It will help get your bowels moving. This will relieve the pressure on your abdomen."

Cec stared at him intently as if trying to discern his credibility.

"Cecile?" Choy said quietly, leaning forward.

"Yes," she said, barely moving her lips.

"Yes to the Octreotide?"

"You can try."

"Where did it go?" Cec was rummaging about on her bedside table. "I thought it was here."

We were alone in the room.

"What are you looking for?"

"Anne Lamott."

"*Traveling Mercies?*"

Cec nodded, looking around the room with a furrowed brow.

I pulled her bedside table closer. Anne Lamott's *Traveling Mercies* wasn't there. Cec began tidying, stacking empty plastic cups, lining up tubes of ointment. "Is it on the floor?"

I was already walking around the foot of her bed to the far side, the narrow strip of floor between the bed and the windowsill.

There was a stack of books on her small night table. On top of the books sat the telephone. Beside the telephone, a bouquet of flowers in a wide-neck vase. I moved the phone off the stack of books.

"They've gone off in a corner and multiplied," I said as I lifted the books. She looked at me quizzically. I don't think she heard me.

It was amazing to me that she could look so childlike (that innocent crinkle of question in her brow) and in the same moment measurably older (sallow skin, the dull gaze of incomprehension).

Grisham's *The Broker* in hardcover was on the top of the pile of books. I picked it up.

Hardcover. Cec never bought hardcover. When did she buy this?

I tried to think back. Probably in an airport, on one of her trips. I wondered what she was thinking when she picked it up off of the shelf? What propelled her to buy it? In hardcover. The pain in her stomach? *Should I have noticed? Was it a sign?*

I set *The Broker* back on her night table. At the bottom of the stack of books, I found *Traveling Mercies*.

"Why would it be here?" I pulled it out and handed it to Cec.

"One of your rare inspirations to clean up."

"Your table gets so cluttered," I said. She was probably right. My interest and energy for keeping her small hospital room tidy was mild and sporadic. Each morning after the lab tech had been by to collect blood, and the morning nurse had come in to make sure that Cec was still exhibiting discernible vital signs, Cec would invariably say, "How does this place get so messy?" or "Doesn't the clutter bother you?"

My body would tense at her accusation. I'd nod, and murmur, and remain sitting. I needed to know that I could make a decision and it would have an effect, even if it was a negative effect.

I handed *Traveling Mercies* to Cec and she laid it on her lap. I set the rest of the books back on the night table, thinking as I did that maybe I should find another place for them. I lifted the vase out of the metal pail to see if the flowers needed water. They looked fine.

I felt a hand on my thigh. Cec. Her hand moved to the inside of my thigh. I stood still. She squeezed, gently, no mistaking her intent. My body responded, instinctively, the expansive warmth of arousal. I stood with my eyes fixed on the flowers. I could have looked at her. I could have let her pull me toward her.

We hadn't made love in years. For three years, she'd been turning away from me in bed, moving away from my kiss. She said she didn't want to lead me on. Now that she was dying—her breath sour, her eyes yellow—now she was reaching for me? Why? Was she offering me a consolation prize now that her time was up?

A part of me wanted to take her hand even as I felt the blush of outrage creep up my neck. All those nights she'd rolled away from me in bed, all those times she'd accused me of flirting, said I'd sleep with anyone given half an opportunity. I never had.

I pulled a dead flower off the bouquet, then another. I

kept my face turned away, the muscles in my legs stiff, my feet planted.

Her hand dropped away.

I walked past the cards standing on their thin edges on the light-soaked sill. When I reached the end of her bed, I turned to her. Her eyes were closed. She was holding *Traveling Mercies*, loosely, with both hands.

Wednesday, March 16

Cec woke in the middle of the night with a cry of pain. Lorraine must have been on her way into the room. She was at Cec's side before I'd managed to extricate myself from my blankets.

"You want ten?" Lorraine said checking the IV monitor.

Cec nodded.

"I'll be right back."

I took Cec's hand. She squeezed. I closed my eyes, bowed my head. All I could do was hold her hand.

"Aaaahhhh—"

"Can I get you something?"

"She coming?"

"She'll be here—" And then Lorraine was back and I moved out of the way so she could give Cec the shot.

"Ten?" Cec asked.

"Ten," Lorraine said.

"When can I have more?"

"Two hours. If it's bad, maybe an hour."

Cec's jaw was clenched.

"Do you meditate?" Lorraine put her hand on Cec's shoulder. "That can help."

Cec looked startled. She said something that sounded like, "Cockatoo on the peaches."

"Babe? I'm right here."

"She isn't straight that way."

"You're in the hospital, remember?"

"Not under the mattress." She shook her head.

"In the hospital. I'm right here with you."

"It's unfriendly, the way you turn."

"I'm right here. I won't leave you."

"To go to the bathroom?"

"Do you know where you are?"

"Not in the sacred."

Her eyes closed.

My cellphone vibrated. I stepped out of the room. Cec looked like she was sleeping, but I couldn't be sure. I didn't want to wake her. I also didn't want to be out of earshot in case she needed me.

It was Tom. He was using his business voice but he sounded nervous.

"You can take whatever time you need," he hesitated, "but if you—do you think you could maybe come in sometime, for a couple of hours?"

"I'll try." I was just outside Cec's door and talking in a low voice. It was comforting to talk to someone from the outside. "I'll try to get away. I'm just not sure when."

"How are you doing?" The concern in his voice caught me by surprise.

"I'm hanging in. Except that sleep deprivation does not agree with me."

"Are you sleeping there?"

"In her room, on a cot that's too short."

"Well listen, if you'd prefer Chinese water torture…"

"Don't worry, I'll call you. But forget the water, just bring your gun."

"For you or her?"

"Oh, me first." I gave a rueful laugh. "Well, actually I think I'd have to give her dibs."

"That bad?"

"Beyond that bad."

I heard what sounded like a ruffle of blankets from inside Cec's room and peeked in. She was pushing back her blankets. It looked like she was trying to crawl out of bed.

"I have to go. I'll call you later."

I walked back into her room. "You need to go to the bathroom?"

Cec stopped shoving at her blankets. "Who were you talking to?"

"Tom."

"You sounded pretty cheerful for someone whose partner is dying."

"Cheerful?"

"I heard you laughing. That's not showing much respect!"

My cheeks were instantly hot. Anger. And guilt. Stupid guilt! I pressed my lips shut. If I said anything I would cry. Or tell her to go to hell.

I don't know his last name, just his first name: Christian. The Danish photojournalist. I can't find his address, or a phone number, not in any of her address books, not even an email.

I ask Sheila whether she has his contact information.

"Who?"

"The guy that Cec was with, after Jens."

Sheila shakes her head, "Cec never talked about a Christian."

"Not even when you went to visit her in Denmark?"

"Never."

"But…she said she was with him for seven years."

"I don't know. She was very private."

"I can't find anything—not a letter, not a business card—and now you don't know. I'm beginning to wonder…"

Why would she talk about going over to his house and cleaning out his fridge? That was so mundane. It made him seem like a real person, which made me more willing to accept that she had gone with him to the emperor's coronation ball in Japan. She'd shown me a small inkpad and a stamp with the Japanese word for happiness, or luck, I can't remember which. Each of the guests had received one.

Or maybe she'd bought it in a souvenir shop.

I don't know anymore, and now I can't ask.

I try Googling: CHRISTIAN PHOTOJOURNALIST

I should have included Denmark as a search variable.

Never mind, the second result on the Google list is: Christian Als, Photographer. He's from Denmark. And he has his own website. He is also featured on another website. He's the only "Christian" on the site. But he's too young. Born in 1974.

The Christian I'm looking for will be mid-forties, at least. There is a Hans Christian Jacobsen, also a photojournalist. His website offers very little personal information but it says he's been a photojournalist since 1990. That's promising. His photo blog is even more interesting. The pictures are evocative. There's a vibrancy in the light, a kind of movement.

I email him:

> Hello, my name is Lyn. I live in Calgary, Canada, and I'm wondering whether you are Christian, the Danish photojournalist who knew Cecile Kaysoe? She mentioned a photojournalist named Christian but never gave a last name. I'm wondering whether you are that person?
>
> Lyn

He doesn't reply right away.
Days go by.
I give up.
Then I receive this:

> Dear Lyn,
> I do not remember anyone by that name…sorry! I hope you will be successful in your search. There are not many photojournalists by that name…Hans Christian

He sounds kind, and sincere. I am disappointed. I wish it were him. I like his photos, and then I would have confirmation that he wasn't a fabrication.

I've also been looking for evidence that Cec had her pilot's license, like she said she did, but I haven't found it in her papers. I've never seen a picture of her in a cockpit at the controls, just one photo of her and Jens standing in front of a small twin engine. She said they co-owned the plane with another couple. The picture doesn't prove she ever flew a plane.

I wish I'd asked more questions.

"They're gonna give me a car wash." Cec beamed up at me from her recliner. Had the circles around her eyes grown darker or was it just the sunlight on her face that made her cheeks look paler? "Jessie said she would. I don't even have to stand up."

Cec liked that they could wheel her in, strip her down, and scrub her clean while she sat there—a naked princess in all her bloated glory. I liked it that she liked it and that I didn't have to try to help her in that impossibly small shower stall.

She hated smelling sick. Loathed it. With her uncanny nose, she knew better than anyone the sour odor that emanated from her skin—a faint waft of sick breath, unwashed hair, dried blood.

When they rolled her back into the room, the smell of flowery soap wafted in with her. She gave me a smug look of satisfaction.

"What am I going to wear?"

"You want to be in your bed or the recliner?"

"You need to blow-dry my hair. And figure out what I'm going to wear tomorrow, for my appointment."

Finally, we were going to see the oncologist at the cancer centre. Her appointment was at eleven. She would have to to be ready by nine.

Did she really want me to blow-dry her hair? I was awkward with a blow-dryer. Maybe Lorraine or Jessie could do it. I opened her closet door.

"So, what are you going to wear?" I held up a pale-blue

pajama top and matching bottoms. "How about these?" I'd bought them for her a few days earlier.

"No," she shook her head, "the bottoms are too small."

"Already?" I shouldn't have been surprised. Her belly had continued to balloon.

"And that top is too big." She pointed at a set of dark-grey flannel pajamas. I'd bought them in the men's department to get bottoms that were large enough.

"You could put on the dark-grey bottoms with…" I searched through the pile of pajamas on my cot. "Here. You could put this under the top." I held up a pale-grey, long-sleeved shirt.

Cec was the one who had an eye for size and colour.

"Go look on the bed," she'd say when I got home from work.

"What did you buy me?"

"A surprise. Go look."

On the bed I'd find a large shopping bag with several pairs of pants, a dress shirt for work, flannel shirts for chores, a sweatshirt, underwear. She had this uncanny knack for buying me clothes that fit and, most of the time, clothes that I liked.

"Let's see." She held the pale-grey shirt up against herself.

"The dark-grey flannel could go over top. Leave it unbuttoned and roll up the sleeves."

We didn't bother trying the pants—too much work to get her upright and into them—but I helped her out of her nightie and pulled the pale-grey shirt over her head, like helping a child dress. I left the dark-grey top unbuttoned, rolled up her sleeves, and handed her the mirror.

She studied herself with the same squint-eyed appraisal as if she had just put on a business suit.

She asked me to find her perfume.

"One last shred of vanity," she said as she rubbed her wrists together.

I was perched on the edge of the recliner, the FOR SALE papers on my lap on top of a book. I was filling in the makes and models of our three vehicles, the one dollar that I would pay Cec for each of them, glad I'd had the presence of mind to bring copies of vehicle registrations and insurance.

"A choir," Cec said.

"What?" I looked up. I hadn't realized she was awake.

"I want a gospel choir at my service," she said.

"And what would you like them to sing?"

"Amazing Grace."

"Where would you like the service?"

"With Ellen and Mom—"

"At Queen's Park?"

She nodded. Her eyes clouded over, and then they closed. I had more questions, and not just about arrangements. But there wasn't enough time. There would never be enough time. When she was gone, I'd be left with the remains of our life together—with the farm, and the animals, and a pile of unanswered questions.

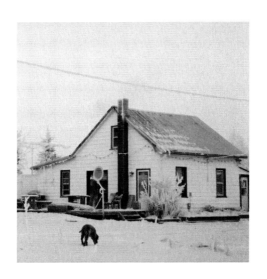

"Can't get a waybill to that port from here"

This was the day Cec had been waiting for with a flicker of residual stubbornness. The cancer centre was on the other side of the city and patient transport needed time for transit and paperwork.

I helped Cec to the bathroom to wash up. We had decided against washing her hair but she wanted me to wet it down, put some gel in, tease it with my fingers. Neither the gel nor the teasing made any difference. Her hair remained dull, lifeless. Cec brushed blush onto her cheeks but decided against mascara or eye shadow. She didn't have the energy.

I was worried about the wear and tear on Cec, whether they would give her enough morphine for the road, what the gyne-oncologist would say.

"When is Allie coming with your morphine? They're going to be here any minute."

"Relax!"

I wanted to find Allie, make sure she hadn't forgotten about the morphine. Instead I said, "No bowel movement this morning?"

"Nope."

"Do you need to go?"

"Why are you so jumpy?"

Cec had become her version of "regular" over the last few days, often producing a small stool mid-morning.

"I don't want you to have to go while we're in transit."

"I'll be fine. Settle down."

I sat down in the recliner. My knees jiggled.

"Relax!" she said again, in that tone I'd heard so many times.

Allie arrived with Cec's morphine injection moments before two six-foot male paramedics in dark blue arrived with a stretcher on wheels. They lowered it to help Cec get on. When they raised it up again I said, "She can't lie back!"

"I'm fine," she said in a low growl.

They raised up the back of the gurney so we were face to face, then rolled her down the hall, one large man at each end. We stopped at the nurses' station.

The nurses already knew. Of course they knew. If they hadn't read it in the chart, they'd seen it come across a computer screen or heard from Allie. Someone got Cec's chart for the paramedics. Three pairs of eyes followed us from behind the nurses' station. Two more stood near the doorway. One emerged from a room and waited while we passed. They all knew what was coming. Their professional sadness expressed itself in silence, a kind of standing at attention.

The paramedics took Cec down the back elevator, along a deserted hallway, through the Emergency Ward to the ambulances and the patient transfer vehicles. They lifted Cec in and asked whether I wanted to ride up front. No, I wanted to be in the back, with Cec.

I sat beside the paramedic on a narrow bench. He took her blood pressure, checked her vitals, asked about her pain, made notes. I watched where we were going through the back window.

In the transfer van, not long after we left, Cec said she felt as though she had to poop but thought she could hold it. Her brow was furrowed.

We'd been on the road for five minutes when she said, "I gotta go!"

I said to the paramedic, "Do you have a bedpan?"

He looked at me blankly.

"A bedpan! She isn't going to make it!" I was already pulling open Cec's housecoat, searching for the waistband of her pajama bottoms. The paramedic found a pink plastic bedpan. I pulled Cec's bottoms down, awkwardly, and the paramedic shoved the bedpan under her. I hoped it was in the right position.

The van filled with the smell of shit. Thankfully, miraculously, all of it hit the pan. I could see the relief on Cec's face, and also her discomfort at having a plastic dish under her. But to remove it would likely have meant getting shit on her, or me. There was so little space to manoeuvre.

"Leave it there," Cec said through a clenched jaw. I wanted the driver to drive faster. Couldn't he put on his flashing lights and siren?

"I'm so sorry," Cec said trying to wave away the smell.

"Forget it. I'm just glad there was a bedpan."

"I feel like such a fool." Mortification in her eyes.

"No, don't."

When we got to the cancer centre, they rolled her down the hallway, into the elevator, and into the reception area where all the cancer outpatients were sitting and waiting for their appointment. The paramedic went to find a nurse. The nurse went to see about an examination room. The seconds ticked by slowly. Didn't these people realize how much pain she was in? She still had the bedpan under her.

We had to wait much longer than my impatience and acute awareness of Cec's discomfort could tolerate. I bit my tongue. I made myself stand stone still beside the stretcher. Cec was keenly aware how much she needed the help of these people, even when they moved slowly. I knew that she wouldn't want me to make a scene.

The nurse came back. She'd found a room. The paramedics wanted their stretcher back. They rolled Cec into an exam room so the nurse could help her get off the bedpan and clean her up. The nurse was dressed in pink. She had a soft voice and kind eyes. Once the bedpan had been extricated, the paramedics rolled Cec out into the hall again and the nurse helped her off the stretcher and into the bathroom. The paramedics took the stretcher. The nurse found a wheelchair for Cec so she wouldn't have to walk the twenty steps back to the exam room. I was sent upstairs to admitting to get her registered.

Registered? I had to get her registered? She'd been in the Calgary hospital system for two weeks. Couldn't the hospital have sent her records over? Couldn't the cancer centre have registered her before she showed up in their waiting room?

I had imagined that we would roll Cec right into a room, talk with the doctor, and roll her out again, back to a waiting vehicle. But apparently no one could talk with her until she became a number. I handed Cec's chart across the counter and waited. Half an hour went by. A woman called my name, walked me into her office, asked a few questions. I waited, again, wondering about the other people in the waiting room. *Sick themselves? Dying? Waiting with others who were sick, dying? How much pain were they in?*

When I finally got back, Cec was in an examination room. She was sitting in a chair and talking with a nurse who was asking her for her whole story, from the beginning: family history, family illnesses, first symptoms, treatment, medications, current level of pain. Until that moment, I'd had this idea in my head that all the background information was in Cec's chart and that anyone who needed to could read her story there. Somehow I had expected that the gyne-oncologist would walk in and get down to the business of her cancer, treatment, prognosis.

Cec was containing her expression of pain, but I could see that she was barely holding it together.

She asked for morphine and the first nurse, the one dressed in pink, went to get an order. She returned with two tablets. Cec wanted an injection. She told the nurse about her butterfly; they could inject into that site. The pink nurse pursed her lips and left again.

The other nurse, the one who had taken Cec's history, came back to say that Cec would need to change into a paper gown for an exam. Cec looked at me in disbelief. *An exam? Didn't everyone here already know her status? What more was there to be discovered by poking around?*

I was about to object, but Cec squeezed my arm. "Just do it," she said.

I helped her take off her clothes. To get her pants off, I lifted her to a standing position. She leaned on my shoulders, heavily, while I pulled her pants down. Her legs shook as she stood.

"Rub my bum," she said. There was a deep groove where the bedpan had dug into her skin. "It's numb."

I massaged the red ring. She said, "I have to sit."

A young woman knocked, then entered. She was wearing a white lab coat and stylish glasses. She was an intern, she said. She needed to ask some questions.

Cec and I looked at each other. *Where was the gyne-oncologist?*

"Where did you first feel pain?" The intern looked like she was in her twenties, her pen poised over her clipboard.

"The other nurse already asked this." I had to say something.

"I need to review her medical history."

"But we've already gone over and over all this. Can't you see that she's in a lot of pain?"

"This is part of the procedure," she said. "I'll need to do an exam."

"You're kidding!" She wasn't the oncologist.

Cec grabbed my arm. She could see that I was about to lose it. I looked at her. She shook her head and whispered, "If we have to."

We were at the mercy of the institution and Cec was prepared to do whatever she had to do to reach the wise woman with the magical potion that Cec was hopeful might save her.

The intern asked a few more questions. I glared at her the entire time, shooting beams of fury into the side of her head. I think it helped. I'm pretty sure she skipped a bunch of the questions on her list.

"Okay," she put down her clipboard, "I'll need you to get up onto here."

She helped me get Cec up onto the exam table. Cec didn't utter a sound.

"She can't lie down." I was growly as a mother bear. There was a bit of a commotion as the intern and the pink nurse tried to figure out how to raise the back of the table so Cec could sit up and lean against it. The intern listened to Cec's heart and took her blood pressure. Then she wanted Cec to lie back, put her feet in stirrups.

"I can't lie on my back," Cec said in a small voice. "Please don't make me."

The intern wasn't about to budge. She was determined to have her go.

"Should I stay or go?" I asked Cec.

"Stay. Face toward me." She pulled me to her. "Put a sheet over my legs," she said to the intern.

I held Cec's hand while they lowered her until she was lying flat. Cec squeezed my hand. I could barely stand it.

The pink nurse was on the other side of Cec. Her eyes were apologetic. She knew. Cec groaned. Then she cried out. The intern stopped, pulled off her plastic gloves. The pink nurse helped Cec sit up again.

The intern said she would be back. Cec remained on the table, waiting.

We never did see Dr. Lillian Denton.

A small, balding man in a grey suit came into the room

with the young intern trailing behind. I don't remember his name. He looked at her chart. He'd obviously been debriefed by the intern.

He said that he needed to have a look for himself.

"But she just did an exam!" I pointed at the intern.

"I'll need you to lie back," the man said to Cec.

"It's very painful for her to lie flat."

"This won't take long."

I sat facing Cec. I held her hand tight. I couldn't look at her. This time, she began moaning, loudly, almost immediately. He barely examined her at all.

"You can raise her up again," he said to the pink nurse. He peeled off his latex gloves and consulted Cec's chart as he perched on the edge of a stool.

"The cancer is advanced, and very aggressive. A cancer this aggressive is rare." He paused, folding his fingers together. "There isn't much that I can offer you in terms of treatment. Chemo might be an option but it would be very hard on you. You are in a weakened state already and the negative side effects could be potentially devastating. If I thought that chemo was a good option, I'd be selling it hard, but I'm not."

He paused.

"Are there any other options?" This from Cec.

"Our only other option at this point would be an experimental drug. I can offer no guarantee that it would have any effect."

Cec would be offering herself up as a guinea pig. He didn't use the words "guinea pig," but his meaning was clear.

Cec looked at me. "What do you think?"

She was considering this? I was surprised, but not really. Chemo, even an experimental drug, represented her last hope.

"I think chemo would be very hard on you."

She nodded. "But it might help."

"You can give it some thought," the oncologist said. "If you decide to go ahead, we'd want to start next week."

"Would I have to come here?"

"Not necessarily. You could receive treatment where you are."

"I need to think about it. And talk to Lyn."

He nodded. "You'll also want to consider your care options. If you decide against chemo, home care would be a possibility, or a hospice. There are a number of good hospices in the city."

The nurse in pink said, "I can get you some information to take with you."

The man in grey began gathering himself to go. I had one last question, the most important one, the one we'd been waiting to ask.

"Uh—" I held up my hand. He looked at me.

"What about prognosis? I mean, if she doesn't do the chemo, how much time?"

He looked at Cec and said, "That will be up to you." He spoke softly but without hesitation. "Get your affairs in order, your will and any final wishes. Talk with your family. When you are ready, when you've had enough, you will go very quickly. I don't know exactly how long. The cancer is advanced. Maybe days, maybe weeks. It's different for each person. Much depends on your will to live. This really is up to you."

It was evident that he was giving us a hard truth as clearly and gently as he could. He could see that Cec was running on the fumes of willpower. Her resolve had been fuelled, until this moment, by a small reserve of hope.

The pink nurse handed me brochures about support groups for family and friends of the terminally ill. She pointed to information on grief support.

"I know it's hard to think about this," she said. "They offer an important service."

I couldn't stop the tears. The nurse handed me a tissue, and another. Cec was still on the exam table, sitting up. I sat down on a stool beside her, my head level with her elbow. She put her hand on the back of my neck.

"Thank you," Cec said to the man in grey. She was sincere.

He nodded and left the room.

"Could we have a moment?" Cec said to the pink nurse.

"I'll call patient transfer and let them know you're ready."

I sat with my head bowed, the side of my face resting against Cec's leg. She ran her fingers up the back of my neck into my hair as I tried to snuffle back tears.

"At least we can begin the grieving process together," she said. I looked up at her. Her eyes were wet, the first tears I'd had seen her cry since I'd brought her into Emergency. It was the first time she let me cry without reprimand.

I wanted to sit there forever. I didn't want her to lift her fingers from my neck. Long after her death, I could still feel her fingers massaging my scalp.

The nurse returned. It was time to get Cec back into her clothes for the return trip. Cec asked for another shot of morphine.

The nurse went off to get permission and I helped Cec off the exam table and back into her clothes. This time I put a diaper on her, just in case.

Two different paramedics came with a stretcher and helped Cec onto it, lifted the back up. They wheeled her into the waiting area again, into a stall along the side with a curtain that could be pulled around. I couldn't make my tears stop. The woman at the reception desk brought us a box of tissue.

"She's having a meltdown," Cec said to the paramedics, apologetically, as though she was the mother and I was her child. Cec pulled me closer and wiped my wet cheeks with the heels of her hands. There was tenderness in her voice, in her touch. Her gentleness had a calming effect.

I didn't think it in that moment but later, looking back, I knew her ability to touch with tenderness was one of the reasons I'd stayed. I could sense her capacity for gentleness, even in her tone of annoyance and her cutting criticisms.

The ride back was quiet. I got my tears to stop, and I was glad to get back to the hospital and up to Cec's room. Each nurse, in turn, looked up as we made our way down the hall. I could see the questions in their eyes. We kept moving.

When we got back to her room, I helped Cec into bed. She asked for the phone. I lifted it off the nighttable and set it on her lap.

"I'm glad to be back here," I said. And I was. Deeply relieved.

"Funny," Cec said, "you're more institutionalized than I am."

Cec talked about her trip to the cancer centre as though she'd been to the opera. She didn't leave out any of the parts including her sudden need to shit in the transfer van, the discomfort of sitting on the bedpan, the stupidly flat examination table, the redundant questions, the multiple pokings.

She called Lora first: "Lyn was in worse shape than I was...I know...yeah...she kind of lost it...no, not a lot of fun...but it's over...uh-huh...a nurse, an intern, and then the doctor...exactly the same."

To Sheila: "An experimental drug...I said no...yeah...that's right...they didn't say...yeah...uh-huh...stupid system... an intern first...I guess they have to practice on someone."

"Would you like a foot massage?" Lorraine had just given Cec her shot of morphine.

"Maybe later. I need to just lie here for a bit."

"You can let me know. I'll send someone in whenever you're ready."

Lorraine remained standing. She shifted to her other foot. I could tell she wanted to ask. Then she did. "How'd it go today?"

Cec's eyes were closed.

"Tough trip," I said.

Cec opened her eyes, "I was hoping for one more season of golf, but it looks like that's not in the cards."

Lorraine sent Curtis in to give Cec a foot massage.

"Ready for some pampering?" He was carrying a basin of warm water.

"Bring it on." Cec beamed at him.

"Didn't I tell you they give me the easy jobs? You okay to sit in one of those chairs?"

"For you, anything."

"This is not about me. It's all about you."

"Put me in the chair."

I helped him move Cec from the bed to one of the hard-backed chairs.

"Aaaahhhh…" An exhale of pleasure as Curtis lifted her swollen feet into the water. He knelt on the floor and massaged her calves.

"I heard you had a hard day," he said, his head bowed.

"Not exactly the best day of my life."

"How does that feel?" he asked, splashing water on her calves.

"Lovely," she murmured, with a little smile.

"You going to fall asleep on me?"

"No." Her eyes closed.

"Tell me a story, if you're not too tired, something about your life."

I wasn't sure she would respond.

"Hafta think." The words were barely audible. After a few moments, she said, "I lived in Denmark."

"You did?" He looked up. "Do you speak Dutch?"

"Danish," I said. "We both do."

Curtis swivelled his head to look at me. "You do? Are you Danish?"

"No, but we both lived there. Not at the same time."

"I was married to a Dane." This from Cec.

Married? I saw the question in Curtis' eyes. He didn't ask. He just said, "Say something in Danish."

Cec smiled at me. *"Jeg elsker dig, meget højt."* (I love you, very high)

"*I lige mode*," I replied. (In like manner, or likewise)
"What did you just say?" he wanted to know.
"I said, 'How are you?'" Cec said.
"And I said, 'Fine, thank you.'"
"Say it again."
"You want to hear my story?"
"Tell me." Curtis grinned.
"I owned a freight forwarding company in Copenhagen."
"You did?"
"I did, Aeroship, and one day a guy came to see me—"
Had I heard this story before?
"—he asked me whether I knew a Hans Kaysoe."
Curtis was massaging her feet.
She leaned her head back. "World War Two. Hans and Greta Kaysoe, my mother and father-in-law. He was trying to find them." Cec grimaced and leaned forward.
"You okay?" I asked. "Would you prefer the recliner?"
Cec shook her head. "Don't wanna move." To Curtis, "Don't stop." She took a deep breath. "He was a little boy in World War Two. His parents…" a long exhale, "…fled the Nazis. From Poland." She paused. "Came to Denmark." Her eyes closed and she gripped the armrests. "Hans and Greta…"
"Your in-laws hid them?"
"Got them on a boat…to Sweden."
"More morphine?" I asked Cec.
"Wait," Cec held up her hand. "He wanted…to meet them. To…say thank you."
"How old was he when they left Poland?" Curtis asked.
"Six. Or seven."
"And he remembered their names?"
"My father-in-law was dead."
"Did he meet your mother-in-law?"
Cec nodded. "They both cried. He kept saying he owed her…his life."

I'd never heard this story before.

How many more stories were there, I wondered, that I'd never heard? That I would never hear?

"That's a wonderful story," Curtis said. "Thank you."

"Okay. Morphine," Cec said. "Now."

The nine o'clock announcement came over the hospital PA system. Visiting hours were over. All visitors were asked to please leave the ward.

The nurses didn't usher visitors out or do any kind of physical check. The ward doors remained open. The end of visiting hours was marked by footsteps in the hallway and a momentary surge in conversation.

It felt to me as though the steel doors were clanking shut. Locked down. Locked in.

"Hafta go," Cec was in her recliner, propped with pillows, legs raised, ready for the night.

"You have to go?"

"You," she pointed at me, "hafta go. Home."

"But I'm not a visitor."

"Hafta sleep."

"I'm staying here with you."

She gave me a look of non-comprehension.

"The nurses said I could, remember?"

"Oh yes, that's right," she said, nodding, as though I'd jogged her memory.

I slept fitfully. I'd drop away into dream, then jerk awake. I'd open my eyes whenever a nurse came in, or when the gears in Cec's hospital bed would grind. The quiet would settle again, and I'd fall back into agitated dreaming. My dreams were never of the outside world. My dreams were the half-lucid contortions, the hum, the boredom, the crisis of this room.

The next morning I said to her, "Last night you told me

that I should go home. Did you mean that? Did you want me to leave?"

"Oh no." She smiled and patted my arm. "No, of course not."

Friday, March 18

No more tests. No treatment. We had reached the end of the line. Except that she hadn't yet come to a complete stop and no one could tell us when that would happen.

"She declined treatment," Choy said, as though to remind me.

"There weren't any good options."

"I'm sorry," he said, "I know this is hard."

It was happening too fast. I had to remember to breathe. If I didn't remind myself, I would find myself holding my breath.

Lora hadn't arrived yet. I think she knew that others were coming today. Now that the verdict was in, there was a steady stream. Cec's niece and nephew had come from Long Island, and her brother from Germany.

I stood at Cec's doorway and regulated the flow of visitors. No more than two at a time.

"Please be very quiet. If her eyes are closed, just sit with her. She needs to sleep."

Cec had stipulated that she didn't want anyone from her work to visit. If any of her colleagues showed up, I was under strict orders not to let them in. I was standing guard to make sure no one slipped past.

In the moments when there were no visitors, I would lower myself quietly into a chair beside her bed. When she opened her eyes, I'd watch her mind processing with effort. If she tried to talk, her words often came out in a jumble.

She had flashes of coherency but mostly she seemed to float along on waves of disjointed thought. Along both her arms were brown blotches. The first had appeared several days before. Since then, they had multiplied rapidly.

A new nurse had come into the room the other day, one I hadn't seen before. Cec looked liked she was sleeping. The nurse stood there for a minute, then she whispered, "Is this your grandmother?"

I shook my head. I hoped Cec hadn't heard.

"Your mother?"

"My partner." I glared at her.

"Oh."

"She needs to sleep."

I stood with an empty cup in my hand staring at the microwave. I knew I should fill the cup with water and put it in the microwave but I just stood there.

"It's not easy to watch them go." I recognized Jessie's voice and felt the warm weight of her hand on my shoulder. "I know. I lost my mother a year ago. It took me a long time. You feel like the sun isn't going to shine again, don't understand how anyone can smile. But then one day the clouds will lift and you'll catch a glimpse of sunlight. It does happen. Takes time." Her voice got soft, "Won't be long now." She spoke gently, "You can see in her eyes. They're yellow. Her fingers and toes are turning blue at the tips. That means her circulation is shutting down. When that starts to happen, it's never long."

I looked at her with the question I knew she couldn't answer.

"I don't know how long. Everyone is different. And some are real fighters. I think she is."

I was sitting with Mom and Dad in the wheelchairs outside Cec's room. One of her sisters was in with her.

"I've been praying for Cec," Mom said. "And for you."

"I know. Thank you."

Mom sat with her hands clasped. "I've had an experience that I've never had before," she said.

I waited.

"I think I understand a little better what it's like, for you."

"What do you mean?"

"When someone is sick or dying, they are listed in our church bulletin under Prayer Requests, and they are prayed for from the front." She paused, twisting a tissue. "They know, the people in church, that she is dying, but they don't pray for her from the front. They don't say that they won't. They just don't."

"Have you asked them to?"

"I haven't had to before. I shouldn't have to. It's as though asking for this is somehow not allowed."

"Prayer is prayer, Mom. It doesn't have to happen from the front."

"I know. I just didn't expect this."

I hugged Mom goodbye in the hallway just outside Cec's door. She held me tight. Tears again. I squeezed my eyes to try to stop them.

"You have to go," I loosened my arms from around her but she didn't let me go. We stood face to face, still in embrace.

"I wish I could stay with her and send you home to bed."

"Me too." I was desperate to sleep in a real bed with Noddy bunched up against my legs.

I let her hug me again. More tears.

"What can I do?" Mom asked.

There was nothing she could do. Except give me a tissue. She rummaged in her purse. She always had a tissue, usually rumpled, sometimes with a smudge of lipstick.

"I have to go back to her," I said as I dried my eyes, blew my nose.

"I know, sweetie."

I couldn't look her in the eyes or the tears would start again. She wanted to put her arms around me, but I couldn't let her. I caught hold of her hand and squeezed. She was on the verge of saying that she wished I could be her little one again, that she wished she could take me in her arms and rock me to sleep. This is what my mother wishes when she feels helpless.

But she didn't say it. She said, "Call me if you need anything. Doesn't matter what time."

I turned toward the wide steel door. Mom remained standing in the hall as I pushed the door open. The faint scent of her clung to me—remotely sweet, a hint of Dove soap. After her evening bath, how many times had I heard Mom say, "Good night Dearie" and open her arms for a plush bathrobe hug, her skin still bathwater warm?

The lights were off. I left the door half open to allow in a slice of light. I could make out the outline of Cec's face, her eyes closed, mouth hanging open. The bluish light of the IV screen and the red glow of the CALL button cast faint shadows. The light green fluorescent face of Cec's watch provided a pale indicator of her location. She had taken her other watch off and put this one on the day I brought her in, even though the band was worn and faintly paint spattered. She said she wanted to be able to see the time in the middle of the night.

I worked my way toward my cot, around the recliner. Cec's eyes opened. I stopped. Did she see me?

"Are they gone?" she asked in a croaky whisper.

"Yes, they're all gone."

"I didn't like the circus."

"What?" I leaned closer.

"The magpies make so much noise."

"Yes. I know."

"Keep them in the barn," she said and closed her eyes. I stood and watched her, waiting for more. Nothing. She didn't stir. Her respiration was slow.

I lay on my side, eyes closed, breath shallow, counting the beats between her breaths. I saw Sanjay's hand at the level of my eyes, his fingertips dipping abruptly, his hand dropping. She could tip. Over that edge. At any moment.

I have to keep reminding myself that she's not coming back. Not ever. It's like some kind of black magic. One minute she's complaining about the pillow behind her back and the next her breathing has stopped.

Marion was right. I'm not ready for this.

I still expect to see the hump of her asleep beside me in bed, or the covers pushed back and the shape of her pressed into the sheets. If I close my eyes I can feel the rise and fall of her breathing beside me. There is absence and there is presence.

She is perpetually just around the corner. Her ghost fingers tuck the tag into the back of my shirt.

Sometimes I can feel the sensation of her lying on top of me. Like in the beginning, when we were still new to each other and the farm new to us. Cec would come in from early morning chores and lie down on top of me, the outdoor air clinging to her cheeks, a mingle of fresh alfalfa, damp earth, cuddy cow breath. She'd stretch her wiry frame on top of the blankets on top of me, impossibly heavy, squeezing air from my lungs, her cold cheek against my flushed skin. She'd find my earlobe with her teeth as I struggled to free my arms from blankets so I could wrap them around her and pull her tight. She'd push her lips onto mine with the insistence of an arm wrestle, determined to hold me down, her eyes widening with challenge. I'd squint and pucker, blowing into her mouth. Her body would shudder as she tried to stifle a giggle. I'd open my arms to let her fall against me, the tickle of her hair under my chin, her mouth on my neck.

I miss opening my eyes to her face on the pillow, watching me with one eye and a lopsided grin, "You were snoring."

"No," in a croaky morning voice, clearing my throat, "I don't snore."

Saturday, March 19

Looking back, I feel as though I should have had a clearer sense that she didn't have much time left. I guess I did, in a way.

When I called Doreen I said, "She's fading."

Each time Cec inhaled—struggling to pull air into her lungs—I breathed with her, pulling hard.

It seemed that she was letting herself lean on me, of necessity, not her first choice, but she was finding that I was dependable, and able to bear up. I got the sense that I was her anchor, tethering her, however tenuously, to her remaining moments on this Earth. She had me all to herself. She was my sole focus. I think she could feel that and it helped her relax into a certainty she hadn't felt from me, ever, up to this point.

The surprise for me was her comfort with her own vulnerability, and her trust. I was experiencing the potential I had always sensed existed, in her and between us—her capacity for gentleness, kindness, surrender.

This was part of the reason I had kept deciding, again and again, to stay. I'd seen this potential. The gentle rhythm of our existence, confined to this blue-walled room, was a small consolation, a confirmation that I hadn't been completely crazy to stay. If I'd left I wouldn't have been able to be here, beside her, to know this, to live within this gentler, kinder way of being together for however many moments we had left.

She wasn't in pain, or at least she didn't seem to be.

When Lorraine came to ask whether she needed morphine, Cec waved her away.

She slept. Sometimes she woke. There were stretches, some lasting as long as ten or fifteen minutes, when she was perfectly lucid, fully in charge of her faculties.

"I think you could get about $250,000 for the farm," she said, out of the blue. She was in her bed, sitting up. Her mind was clear. I could see it in her eyes.

"I'm not going to sell the farm." What I realized in that moment but didn't say was that the farm was everything that I would have left of her, of who we were together, and though I didn't know what the distant future might hold, I knew, without a doubt, that I would hold on to the farm like I was holding on to these final moments with her.

Her imprint was all over the farm. She would always be there for me—the energy of her, including her potential to wound, but also her zest for adventure. We'd lived like pioneers on the land, facing the challenges of the unknown. She'd understood how to propel me along. The momentum of her would keep me going, at least for a while.

"You're not?" She sounded pleased.

"No. I can't imagine…"

"What will you do with it?" I could tell she was thinking about all the pieces of our life together and arranging them in a new configuration that was built around me. I couldn't help wondering whether she was feeling the separation from what she once had, the person she was, our life together. Or whether, in her semi-rational, drug-fogged state of mind the farm was with her, immediate, the animals all around her. She seemed completely unrattled, unconcerned that she couldn't go home, would never go back to the farm again.

"I'll keep the small animals," I said, "the chickens, rabbits, goats, maybe a couple of horses." The cows were already gone.

"The llamas?"

"I don't know about llamas."

"And the dogs?"

"The dogs aren't going anywhere."

We went for a walk, me pushing Cec in the wheelchair, slowly, her eyes closed, head falling backwards. The back of her head bumped rhythmically against my belly as I pushed her along the main hallway.

"When is everyone coming?" she asked.

"Lora said she'd come tomorrow."

Her eyes were closed, eyelids yellow, every muscle in her face slack. I was humming "How Great Thou Art" under my breath. On the few occasions when we'd found ourselves in church, each of us holding one half of the hymnal, she'd lean in toward me. My ability to hit the right notes helped her to stay on key. I'd thought my humming might be calming for her, a connection point for her morphined mind to hold fast to. But again, as had so often been the case in our eight and a half years, I was wrong.

"Don't!" She flapped a hand at me. "Not that song!"

I stopped humming, wondering what was going on behind her closed eyes.

When her eyes opened and I could see that she was lucid, I'd ask another question. "Would you prefer to be buried or cremated?"

Her mind turned my question over and over. I'd learned to wait, let her thoughts organize and work their way to her tongue.

"Well," she said, "I guess cremation would be more environmentally friendly."

I waited. Nothing more.

She had asked me, a few days earlier, to find out whether she could be buried with her parents. I called Queen's Park to ask and they said no. Her parents were buried in the veterans' section and it was reserved for veterans and their wives.

"What about the eulogy?" she said. "Have you thought about who you'll get to do it?"

"No."

She was quiet. I waited. Finally she said, "I'm not sure you would be the best person."

Not me? Then who?

I waited.

"A closed service," she said. "Family and close friends only. No one from work. Promise me."

"I promise." I was taking notes. "Anything else?"

"How Great Thou Art."

"Do you know who you want to do the service?"

"Not Jer." Jer was married to Cor, my youngest sister. He was a pastor.

"Why not Jer?"

"I know he'd do a good job but he's family."

Her legs were restless, unbearably heavy, and itchy. She couldn't bend her knees or move her legs without help.

I pushed her blankets aside. Her legs were swollen, the skin taut from stretching to accommodate the build up of fluid. Edema. Her ankles and feet were round as balloons, the skin tight and tinged blue, the deepest blue at the tips of her toes. I curled my hands around one of her thick feet and rubbed.

"My leg…"

I massaged her calf. A fine growth bristled against my palms.

"Lorraine should have given you a shave when you were in the car wash."

"Would you?" Cec asked.

"Shave your legs?"

She nodded. "I need to stand." She reached with both hands and took hold of her upper thigh, tried to lift her leg.

"Here, let me…" I helped her manoeuvre her legs to the side of the bed. "A chair?"

I held her elbows as she lowered her feet to the floor. She leaned against me as we shuffled, in close embrace, until she was positioned in front of the chair. She bent her knees and her body dropped like a stone.

I got a basin of warm water and dug around in her toiletries for her razor and shaving cream.

"Oh, wait. I'll need towels." I spread one towel under the basin and set the other on the end of the bed within reach. I lifted her feet into the water.

"Too hot?" She didn't like her showers as hot as I did.

"It's good." She sat with her arms on the wooden armrests, her back straight, a queen on her throne, and watched as I wet her right calf and lathered. I was kneeling, the basin between my knees, my head and shoulders bowed to reach the water.

Homage, I thought, this simple service.

I felt her hand on the top of my head. Her fingertips massaged my scalp. I couldn't help the tears. I took a deep breath, pressed the razor to her skin and pulled upwards, a long, smooth stroke.

This was one of those moments when I could ask anything.

"Babe?" I wondered whether she could hear that I was crying.

"Yeah."

"I have a question." Why did I say it like that, as though I was in school?

No response.

I looked up.

She was waiting.

"What do you think I should do with my life?"

This wasn't one of the questions I'd had on my mental list. It just came to me, out of nowhere.

I thought she would say that I should plant an organic garden, or write a book.

"I think you should go high up," she said without hesitation, "high up into the mountains, as high as you can go." I had an image of the trail at Lake Louise, the one up to the teahouse. "Get a clear view. Go for the epiphany. I know you've always been afraid of it, but I know you can do it."

No pause. No stumbling. It was as though she had been contemplating this very question, waiting for me to ask.

I stopped shaving. *Epiphany.*

"My death is an opportunity for you," she said.

I looked up at her. *Was she serious?* No tease in her eyes. She meant this. My instinctive response was protest. But deep down I knew she was right.

"You'll get the life insurance," she said, "and the farm. Don't blow it."

I drive onto Hank and Doreen's yard. I haven't called ahead. I need to drive onto a yard unannounced, as though I still belong out here.

Doreen meets me at the front door. Noddy scrambles past her into the house. Hank and Doreen's purebred Collie is never allowed into the house, but Noddy is.

"I just baked cinnamon buns. Would you like one?" The kitchen is warm and filled with the welcoming aroma of fresh baking. Of course I want a cinnamon bun.

"With icing?"

"What's a cinnamon bun without icing?"

Hank is out checking the fields. The minute Doreen sits down at the kitchen table, Noddy is up on her lap.

"I got an offer today," I say. This is why I have come. To tell Doreen.

"Oh? Was it any good?"

"As good as I could have hoped. I've accepted." This admission feels like a confession. There is relief in knowing that the farm is sold, and a nagging guilt. I had told Cec I would keep the farm. And I had. For three years.

"Can I ask you something?" Doreen says as she licks icing from her finger.

"Sure."

"Was Cec ever married?"

I am surprised. Cec and Doreen had talked regularly, but Doreen had obviously never asked.

"She was. They divorced."

"Is her ex-husband still alive?"

"He passed away several years ago."

"Did she have any children?"

I had a mouthful of cinnamon bun and didn't answer right away. "No children. Two miscarriages."

I waited for her next question, which I thought would be about my relationship with Cec—whether she was my partner. But the question never came.

Maybe the fact that Cec had been married was enough. Maybe Doreen figured she knew what she needed to know. Or maybe it didn't matter.

"Would you like another cinnamon bun?"

"Yes, please."

"I need to sleep tonight." I crouched down beside Cec's recliner, my eyes level with hers. I tried to speak softly. Every movement all day had required effort, thoughts fragmented, words plodding. I had to keep reminding myself to suck air in, blow out.

I tried to focus when Choy came by. His words undulated through the air, swam past me. I was afraid he was saying something I would need to know, for a decision I would need to make. *Would I need to make another decision?*

He said something about keeping her moving.

My body was heavy, my mind light. Choy's words droned, the rise and fall of his intonations. I wondered if it made him feel better, all this talking.

And then I knew, the realization settling in, that he was shoring her up, buoying her with his words, in the same way I had kept on showing up for our relationship, kept on listening, and nodding, even when I knew I needed to leave.

Choy stopped talking. He left.

I got off the cot and knelt beside Cec's recliner.

"I'm going to put in my ear plugs," I said, touching her arm. If you need something, you'll have to call the nurse." Cec nodded. I felt a pang of selfishness. *What if she needed me during the night?*

"The CALL button is right beside you."

What if tonight was the night?

"You need to sleep," she said.

"I do."

"It's okay." She closed her eyes.

"Do you need another blanket?"

No. She formed the word with her lips, but made no sound. I peeled off my jeans, pulled my sweatshirt up over my head. I heard her mumble.

"What did you say?"

"I loved you…"

I crouched down beside her.

"I loved you immensely but not wisely." Her voice was weak but she articulated each word clearly.

Immensely, yes. And not wisely.

"What do you mean by that?" I felt selfish, asking her to say it again, but I needed to be sure.

She took a deep breath. "I loved you big, but not good."

How was she able to think this, to process? Where was she finding the words?

I squeezed her hand. "I loved you too." And I had. But not the way she had loved me. "I'm sorry," I said. And I was.

Doesn't matter how long I stare, she doesn't move, her hands on her stomach, fingers stiffly intertwined. I should have expected this. I've been to enough funerals, seen enough dead people.

Cec's face is chalky white, cold skin clinging loosely to bone. The makeup doesn't cover the bruise under her eye. In fact, the purple has deepened. But the hair stylist did a decent job, better than any of my feeble attempts. I wonder how much Cec hated the result of my clumsy efforts and the restraint it required for her to not say so.

No more clumsy. No more not saying what I really think. No more wondering what that final moment will be like.

And something else:

If she could transition into that other dimension without fear or resistance, then I can too. She allowed me to witness her moments of greatest weakness, which were also her moments of greatest strength. She showed me how to bear pain, and how to surrender. I can live the rest of my life without fearing the end of my life. She was right—she will always be with me.

Sunday, March 20

Cec's eyes fluttered open. "They've all been here," she said.
"You've had a lot of visitors."
"Where did they go?"
"Home. Lora will come again later. Cor and Jer said they might bring Aiden and Jonah."
Her eyes closed again. I leaned back in the recliner.
Mom and Dad brought James, my brother, younger than me by a year-and-a-half. No one said he was coming but suddenly he was standing in front of me, slightly taller, with the same mousey-brown hair as me, same slant of cheekbone. He'd driven through the night, would be leaving again in the morning.

"You asleep?" I heard Cec's voice, dimly, through the fog of almost-sleep.
"Almost." I tipped myself forward. "How are you?"
"Hungry."
"Really?"
"Don't want hospital food." She'd been eating a few mouthfuls per "meal," and keeping it down.
"I could get us take out."
"That Thai place across the street."
"You want anything in particular?"
"Vegetables," she said.
I gathered myself to push up out of the chair. "Babe?"

"Yeah."

"When you said last night that you loved me, immensely—Do you remember?"

She nodded.

"Could you tell me—I mean—I think—what did you mean?"

"I loved you in a way that didn't always let you be who you were." No hesitation, and no recrimination for asking.

"It was my fault too," I said, which sounded so feeble.

"No, Lyn, remember…" I waited. "…the good light."

"The good light?"

"Remember the pos—" She took a deep breath.

"—the positives?" Usually she hated it when I finished a sentence for her. This time she gave a weak smile. That was a positive, I thought. Right at that moment I couldn't think of anything else.

I pulled on my jacket.

"Come here." She reached for me, and I moved closer, unsure what she wanted. She grabbed the ends of my zipper, inserted one side into the other and zipped me up, "There."

"Sanks, eh."

Cec was sitting up. She'd pulled her rolling table close—or maybe Allie had—and was waiting expectantly. "I could smell you coming," she said.

"You must be hungry." I was surprised and pleased to hear the strength in her voice. I almost expected her to hop off the bed and say, "Where's my coat? Let's get out of here."

"Pad Thai," I said, setting the bag on the table in front of her, "and veggies."

"Choy came by while you were gone."

"Did you pretend to be sleeping?"

"I was civilized."

"And what did he have to say for himself?"

"He seemed to be under the impression that he had never explained the benefits of that morphine pump he's so keen on."

"That's because you always have your eyes closed."

"Yeah, I should have kept them shut."

"Probably wouldn't have stopped him." I flipped open the lids of the Styrofoam dishes. I knew that Cec found Choy tiring, but I appreciated his willingness to explain the inner workings of illness and medications and procedures.

"Plastic okay?" I held up a plastic fork ensconced in a plastic wrapper.

"If you open it."

I tore open the wrapping and handed her the fork. Her rolling bedside table was too high for me to sit at. And it was narrow. I'd set the two containers side by side and they took up all the available space. So I ate standing up.

Cec snagged a few noodles and lifted them. I watched, pleased to see the dexterity of her fingers, her apparent desire for food, the blush of colour creeping into her cheeks.

"I told him to bring the pump," Cec said, her forkful of noodles suspended mid-air, "but I don't want it."

"You don't have to."

"I think he thinks…" She was chewing.

"You'll be able to top-up faster."

"But I'll be tied to that pole again."

"I know."

"I don't like the pole."

I bit into a lump of tofu, enjoying the burst of heat and garlic. If I'd been sitting on a chair it would have felt as though we were having dinner at home, discussing the day.

"Jer and Cor might come tonight," I said.

"They were here before."

"I didn't think you'd noticed." Cor and Jer had brought Aiden and Jonah for a brief visit that afternoon. Jonah had pointed at Cec: "Why's she sleeping?"

"Shh, Jonah. Auntie Cecile isn't feeling well."

"When will she be better?" Jonah stood on tiptoes.

Aiden had wandered over to the window. "Hey. I see a fire truck!"

"You looked like you were asleep."

"It's my strategy."

It was on the tip of my tongue to ask her whether incoherency was part of her strategy too. Instead I said, "Jer wants to bring his guitar."

"To play?"

I nodded.

"Here?"

"If you'd like him to."

"Will they let him?"

"I asked Allie and she said she didn't think it would be a problem, as long as he plays softly."

"No rock concert?"

"We'll have to close the door."

"When?" She picked a cashew out of the pad Thai.

"They said they'd call. Not as hungry as you thought?"

"I'm not sure I would ever have called it 'hunger.'"

"May I?" I took the Styrofoam dish with the pad Thai and lifted it closer to give myself a better chance at actually getting the noodles into my mouth.

"You have good people in your life," she said.

Had I heard that right? Was she hallucinating? She had only ever made disparaging comments about any of the people in my life. My friends always called at the wrong times, wanted to go out when it wasn't convenient, didn't want to go to places that Cec liked, were too self-absorbed, too emotional, too something. It was always something. But now, with her pain spiking and her mind barely functioning, there was no way to talk about all that, to have the conversation I wanted to have.

"Yes," I said. "I have good people in my life."

The truth of that statement lay in the past. I'd *had* good people in my life. My friends had faded into the background. I had removed myself from so many lives. I had no idea whether any of them would take me back.

Jer and Cor arrived just after seven. Mom and Dad had gone to stay with Aiden and Jonah. Jer leaned his guitar case against the wall.

"Hey, Cec." He had a soothing hospital voice cultivated through the years of being the pastor-on-call. He understood how to tread lightly into a hospital room.

"Hi, Jer," Cec barely turned her head, her strength at a low ebb.

"The boys made these for you." Cor held up two crayon drawings.

"Tell them both thank you. And come over here. How's my boy?"

"He's kicking." Cor pulled Cec's hand to her stomach.

"Alexander," Cec said. She had supplied Cor and Jer with her preferred list of boy names a month earlier. Alexander was at the top.

"Jer wants to name him Andrew. I like Ben."

"She chose the names for the other two," Jer said, "so this time she said I could pick the name."

"Unless it's Andrew." Cor gave Jer an impish grin.

"Alexander would be a good compromise." Cec wasn't about to give up. "You gonna play for me?"

"If you'd like."

"I would."

Jer got out his guitar, began plucking, tuning. I sank into the recliner and closed my eyes. If I tipped back another few degrees and this solitude persisted, I might even fall asleep.

Jer began strumming a hymn I recognized. I couldn't

remember the words. A predictable beat wrapped in a harmony deep enough and wide enough for all tears.

Cec's eyes were closed. She looked like she was floating under a bright sun on a clear, blue sea.

I find this entry in Cecile's medical record, written in the long slanted scrawl of a gastrointestinal specialist whom I remember as basketball-player tall and boyishly blond:

This is a very tragic situation but unfortunately there is nothing that can be done. She has a persistent ileus for a number of reasons but the most important is the diffuse intraperitoneal disease. This is being aggravated by narcotics and the post-op status of the patient. Her exam is typical of this situation. Distended ascites and scant bowel sounds.
My advice: Despite her young age, common sense should prevail. Her lifespan is very limited no matter how heroic one feels obliged to be.

I came into the room one day to find Cec sitting up in bed, a forlorn waif with a deep-purple bruise under her right eye.

She said, "I think I've figured out why we have to get sick before we die."

"Oh yeah?"

"To shed every bit of ego, every last shred of vanity. Look at me! I can't walk by myself. I can't dress. I'm wearing a diaper."

Monday, March 21

I must have slept. It was morning. When I opened my eyes Cec was sitting up in bed, her back to the window. Behind her, the entire frame of the window was filled with swirling cloud.

I thought: *Heaven has come down.*

Then I thought: *Why did I just think that?*

I couldn't shake the feeling that the hand of God (or maybe the finger of God, as in Michelangelo's painting) had reached down to stir up a tumult.

Cec's voice penetrated the sponge of my earplugs, "Dish!"

I scrambled for the basin. She threw up.

Shit! I thought. Damn! We'd had such a quiet, vomitless weekend.

She sat slumped over the basin, one arm hugging her stomach.

This was not going to be a good day.

I yanked out my earplugs, found my glasses, pulled on slippers and a sweater. I took the basin into the bathroom, dumped the contents into the toilet, rinsed it out.

A lab tech knocked as he entered. He set his white plastic box on the floor beside Cec's bed. "Which arm?" He reached for her right elbow.

"Neither!" I said. No one was going to poke her with a needle today. If Sanjay or Steader really needed a blood sample, they would have to convince me.

Cec hadn't lifted her head.

"But…"

"She's in extreme pain!" I glared at him. "She doesn't need anyone sticking a needle in her."

He glanced at the top of Cec's head, then at me, back at her.

"If anyone gives you any grief, you tell them to come talk to me."

"Maybe later?"

"No, not later."

He picked up his case, backed up a couple steps, turned and left.

"Shegum taratara," Cec mumbled. She was flushed, feverish. I went around to the other side of her bed and lowered myself into the recliner. I took her hand. She jerked it away.

"Keela asparga me loop!" An urgent instruction.

Mom arrived to sit with her but I couldn't leave. Cec's pain was spiking. She was getting ten milligrams and it wasn't enough.

I stepped into the hallway to call the Queen's Park cemetery. I had made an appointment to sign the papers but there was no way. I couldn't leave. I sank into a wheelchair in the hallway and dialed. Each time she moaned, my body tightened. Her pain came in waves, like labour.

Lora arrived. Good, I thought, when I saw her walk in.

She'd been given a one-week compassionate leave, she said. She couldn't concentrate anyway.

Lawrence, one of Cec's favorite nurses, padded into the room in his navy-blue scrubs. It was hard to breathe. The room was hermetically sealed. Airless.

Cec didn't want to talk to Choy.

"I'm tired." She waved him toward me.

"How's your pain?"

She didn't answer. He looked at me.

"Nine," I said, tired of pain as a number. "And it spikes. She can't hold anything down."

"We need to get her pain under control—" he put his stethoscope to his ears, "—before we move her."

"Move her?"

"To a hospice."

"Today?"

"When she's stable."

I didn't want them to move us anywhere. We knew the people here, and the routine.

"Cecile?" Choy touched her arm.

She opened her eyes.

"I've ordered the morphine pump. It will help your pain control."

She stared at him blankly.

"I really think it would be best," I said gently.

She closed her eyes.

"It should be here in the next hour or two."

I nodded.

"If you don't want it, you don't have to," Choy said to Cec, "but we'll get it ready, in case."

I couldn't tell whether the clench of her jaw was pain or irritation.

"I'll be back in a little while." Choy turned to go.

I followed him out of the room and pulled the door closed behind me.

"I need to know how long you think she has," I whispered.

"She's deteriorated considerably over the weekend." He paused. "I was going to recommend that we move her to a hospice today but she's too weak. I don't think she'd survive the transport."

"Days? Hours?"

"It's hard to say. So much depends on her will. Could be eight hours, or eighty-eight."

"I think it's closer to eight."

Whenever Mom or Lora were in with her, I'd escape to the hallway and sink into a wheelchair.

Lora appeared in the doorway and motioned for me to come. "She's pouring water on herself."

"What?!" I was up in an instant.

"She poured water on her pillow and put the pillow to her face."

Cec was holding a plastic cup filled with water and ice. She lifted the cup and tipped it toward her head.

"You want some on your head?"

She nodded solemnly.

"Here." I took the cup from her, held it over her head, and poured a thin stream.

Cec shuddered as though she hadn't expected the wet, or the cold. I was instantly sorry.

I walked out of the fish-bowl-blue ward, out through the wide-open double doors of ward 51 into the fleshy pink hallway. I was breathing in small, shallow gulps, dizzy and unsteady on my feet. I reached for the handrail. My stomach was gurgling. Whatever I managed to get down, which wasn't much, ran right through me. I pushed open the door to the public washroom. The sign on the door said: VISITORS.

Was I a visitor? If I couldn't leave?

I closed the door and locked it, stood staring into the mirror. Expressionless eyes looked back at me, puffy, bloodshot. A small white sign reminded visitors to wash their hands.

I washed my hands.

Cec was in the recliner, swaddled in blankets. Lora was sitting beside her, holding her hand. We had agreed, out in the hallway, that we would tell Cec that she could go.

I looked at Lora.

She looked at me.

"You first," I said.

"CeCe?" Lora in her small-girl voice. "CeCe? Can you hear me?"

No response from the recliner. Cec exhaled. Lora and I waited. I was counting. Cec inhaled, sucking hard, shuddering.

"CeCe, it's Lora. I just want to tell you…" Her voice choked. She put her hand over her mouth, swallowed, tried again. "I want to tell you that I love you. And…"

I waited, but she couldn't.

"We want to tell you that it's okay if you go," I said.

"We'll be okay."

"We'll look out for each other."

"We will."

Cec's eyes remained closed. Not a twitch.

Had she heard us? Did she need to?

Marion was sitting with Mom and Dad in the waiting room. They looked up, instantly sober.

"How are you, dearie?" Mom asked.

"Awful."

I wanted to say: "Fucking awful."

I wanted to say: "Thank you for sitting here."

I wanted to say: "Please don't make me go back in there." I wanted to say it all in one word or one blink of my eyes. I didn't have the energy to formulate thoughts, to enunciate.

I didn't sit down. Because I knew I wouldn't get up.

"She doesn't want anyone in there, " Mom said.

I nodded. She didn't want anyone. Except me.

I wanted to say: "Thank you for knowing that."

"I can't breathe," Cec said, in a whisper.

I heard a gurgle from the back of her throat. Then she coughed and motioned for the basin. I held it up. She spit. A brownish blob.

She said "Dish!" again, her hand over her mouth. I got it under her chin just as the vomit came. Her skinny shoulders folded forward as she heaved.

I handed her a glass of water. She rinsed her mouth. Spit. She didn't apologize. The smell didn't make me queasy. I carried the basin to the bathroom and tipped it into the toilet. The odour of vomit clung to me, in my nose, at the back of my throat. I wondered whether the smell had saturated my clothing.

Lora came looking for me. I'd escaped to the hallway again.

"She wants her pillows arranged," Lora said. "I tried to help her but she said that you're the only one who knows how."

Cec was rubbing her back against the pillows.

"7Up," she said.

"But you don't like 7Up."

"Might help."

When I brought the 7Up she took one sip, straight from the bottle—usually she insisted on a cup—and handed it back to me. "Ugh," she turned up her nose.

"I knew you wouldn't like it."

A few minutes later she was throwing up a pinkish liquid fizz.

Cec pointed at the bathroom door. I didn't wait for her to find the words. I went to get her toilet seat on wheels, helped her onto it, rolled her into the bathroom and positioned the rolling seat over the toilet. I stayed standing beside her. She leaned forward, closed her eyes. Nothing. Not even a drop of pee.

"I'm sor…"

"It's okay."

I helped her stand, pulled up her Depends, rolled her back into the room, helped her stand. She stood up straight for a moment on her stiff, thick legs, then bent forward, leaning on the bed with her elbows, face in her hands.

"You want to get into bed?"

She lifted a hand. No.

I waited.

She hunched her back. It looked like she was trying to stretch out her back. Or maybe it was the pain.

She turned her head to look at me.

"Are you still okay with this?" I asked. When we'd talked a couple of days ago, she'd said that she was okay with dying. But this pain—it was too much.

She nodded.

"You sure?"

She pushed herself more upright.

"No waybill," she said.

"What?"

"The papers…you can't get…"

"Can't get—what?" I wasn't sure how to prompt her.

"Can't get a waybill…to that port…from here."

"You mean…"

"Can't get…that port…"

"The destination isn't important."

She nodded.

"It's the journey that matters."
She dropped her head, nodding.

Cec was in a recliner between Lora and me. The light was almost gone from the sky. A dim fluorescent bulb above Cec's bed was flickering, just barely, but enough that my eyes kept watering. I thought about switching it off, but I didn't have the energy to get up.

Choy came by again. He didn't stay long. He said nothing about moving Cec to a hospice, just that the IV pump was ready if she wanted it. Cec didn't respond. He said he'd have Lawrence bring it in and she could decide.

Cec said nothing while he was in the room. As soon as he left, she said, "He can't make me."

"He won't make you, Babe." She was already at ten milligrams. The pump wouldn't let her go higher than that anyway.

"Don't like the sound of that!" Cec said suddenly, sternly.

"It's okay, Cec." Lora stood and moved closer. "You don't have to have the pump. Not today."

Cec closed her eyes again.

Lora squeezed her hand, kissed her forehead. "I love you CeCe." She turned to me. "I'm going to go."

Go? A leap of panic. She was going to go? Leave me alone? I wanted to say: Please don't…Please. Don't leave me.

I sank back into my chair.

"I'll be back in the morning." Lora pulled on her jacket.

The darkness of the night sky outside her window settled on me like a heavy blanket. We were all alone. *What could I say to her?*

Our Father, Who Art in Heaven…

No. Maybe a Bible verse.

*Thou shalt rise up on the wings of an eagle…*No.

…the valley of the shadow of death… More than a shadow, that valley.

"Massage my feet," she said in a whisper that was barely audible.

I would be looking for relief too, I thought. There was no way I could have stood the pain for this long.

I pushed the blankets aside and rubbed her feet. They were swollen, her skin taut and cool to the touch, the tips of her toes a deep purple.

"Remember what the oncologist said? That you could go at any time?" It was all I could think to say. A kind of medical permission.

"I can't just go, Lyn! My heart is too strong. My lungs are too strong." Her voice was still reasonably strong too.

But I needed her to go. I knew I was being selfish but I was teetering—one small nudge away from crying inconsolably and flailing my arms until they wrapped me in a straitjacket and tied me to the bed.

I tucked her foot under the blanket and lifted her other foot. "What do you want? Do you want to go?"

She was quiet for a moment, then, "I want God to fix me. Or shoot me."

She sounded so clear. This wasn't the fading away that Marion had described.

Lawrence was trying to adjust the pillows behind Cec's head. I was on the other side of her bed, trying to help.

I felt as though I was standing on the bottom of a deep pool—the pale fluorescent light, the blue walls swimming. Lawrence's navy blue scrubs and the slow motion of his movements added to the sensation.

I lifted her legs to pull a pillow under her knees. She cried out. Any other time she would have glared at me and said, "You don't know your own strength!" in the same tone as, "You're such an idiot!" Not today. Her head fell back and she shuddered as she sucked in another deep breath.

Mom appeared in the doorway with a plate of food she'd brought from home.

I shook my head at her. "Not a good time."

"I'll be—" Mom pointed down the hall. "I'll wait for you."

"Five minutes." I held up five fingers. Cec's watch said 6:57 p.m.

"Can you help me?" Lawrence said. "Hold her so I can get this one behind her back."

I put my arm around Cec's shoulders and nudged her upright. Lawrence pulled up a pillow that had slid down behind her back. Cec groaned.

It didn't matter how we arranged the pillows. Nothing helped. Morphine was flowing into her bloodstream at a rate of ten milligrams an hour. Not enough for the pain. Too much for mental clarity. Entirely insufficient to end it all.

"Dish!" she said, motioning.

I lifted the dish from the floor and held it under her chin. I heard a gurgling in the back of her throat. She spit. A dark-brown blob.

"Is there more?"

She nodded and cleared her throat. Spit again. Another dark-brown, stringy blob.

"I need air." She was struggling to breathe.

"We need to sit her up," I said to Lawrence. He was across from me, on the other side of the bed.

I held the bowl with one hand and put my other arm around her shoulders, trying to help her sit up so she could breathe more easily.

"Help me! I need to sit her up!" Lawrence didn't seem to understand the urgency. She needed to breathe.

Cec threw up again. Brown liquid. And again. I tried to hold the bowl steady.

More brown vomit. It wasn't really vomit. It was viscera. It was wretchedness.

And then brown liquid poured out of her mouth in a gush, as though a faucet had been turned on.

This vomit didn't stink. It wasn't partially digested stomach matter. This was more ominous. More fatal. I knew, with a strangely calm certainty, that she wouldn't survive this. She couldn't.

Brown liquid began streaming out of her nostrils. Her head fell forward.

Lawrence was pounding the CALL button and yelling for help *now*! I heard the stampede of nurses' shoes.

The basin was full and heavy. The medical report said one litre of stomach contents, but it was at least two litres, maybe even three.

"I think she's gone," I said to Lawrence.

He put his stethoscope to her chest. "I think so too." His eyes were on me. And then the room was filled with nurses.

Someone lifted the basin out of my hands.

"Can I leave now?" I said to no one in particular, the faces a blur.

"Yes," someone said, "you can go."

Mom and Dad were in the visitors' room. My eyes were dry.

"What's wrong?" Mom stood, holding the plate of food.

"I think she's dead."

I open the back door and the hinge creaks. I step across the threshold. Our old farmhouse is silent. This is why I didn't want her to go—this stretched-out silence.

She would come home from work early to do chores and sit at her computer late into the night. For me, she said. She did it for me. She washed the kitchen floor for me. She baked blueberry-cranberry muffins for me. All her energy pointed at me, toward me, with a purpose that held me at its centre.

Even when she would criticize and accuse, it was because of me. My presence made a difference.

I'd clung to the daily demands, the motions I knew by heart—washing dishes, feeding dogs, shovelling frozen cow shit—all those small, never-negotiated and worried-smooth predictabilities; the tilt of her cheeks toward my lips as I leaned over to kiss her good night; the clickety-clack of her fingers on the computer keys; the way she could throw a perfect spiral, the ball motionless in the air until the pigskin burned the heel of my hand; the many small certainties I had come to depend on.

I stand at the patio doors and look south toward the orange glow of city lights against a black sky. The house is cold and I shudder. When the furnace rumbles to life, the floor underneath my feet will tremble.

I am surrounded by a deep and unending emptiness.

I don't want to lie down in an empty bed. I want her to be there. I want her to reach for me. I can still feel the gravitational pull of her desire.

Mom and Dad walked me back down the hall, one on either side. I felt Dad's hand touch my elbow but I moved my arm away. I needed to do this myself.

Cec's hospital room door was closed. A nurse came out carrying an armload of bedding. I asked whether I could go in.

"Not yet," she said. "As soon as they are finished."

I should have stayed with her, I thought. *Why did I leave?* It felt strange to be denied entry. That was my room too.

I sat down in one of the wheelchairs lining the hall. Mom was in a wheelchair on one side, Dad on the other. We sat silent, in a kind of vigil.

Eventually, a doctor—a young woman I'd seen before but had never talked with—came out of Cec's room. She was holding a clipboard against her chest. She stopped in front of us and said, "I'm really sorry. You can go in now."

Mom started to get up but I put my hand on her arm to stop her. "I need to… myself…" She sat back down.

I pushed open the door and realized that I'd been expecting to see Cec propped up in bed like always. But that wasn't how it was. The back of Cec's bed had been lowered. She was lying completely flat, which looked odd. And the bed had been lowered so it was the height of a normal bed. That was doubly odd. A white sheet covered her up to her shoulders. The nurses had cleaned her up but there was still blood crusted under her nose and splatters on her nightgown. Her mouth hung open.

"Babe?" I whispered. I didn't expect an answer, but I sort of did.

It was hard to comprehend. One moment she was moaning and the next, silent.

I crouched beside her.

"I'm sorry," I whispered, to the blanketed shape of her now-silent body. I wondered whether she knew that I had been wishing she could go.

But I hadn't expected... I'd thought there would be a moment, before the curtain fell, when we would know... Or at least that she would know, in the way she always just seemed to know.

I felt strangely peaceful, a calm exhaustion, a numbing disbelief. The hard realization would come later, the next morning, when I opened my eyes to the pale grey light of Mom and Dad's guest room; when I surfaced from a sleep so deep it was like a loss of consciousness. I would open my eyes and suddenly know that she was dead and feel the enormity, and the permanence, of her absence. The understanding would ram itself through me. I'd curl into a ball, barely able to breathe.

But as I crouched beside her, and then sat beside her on the edge of her bed, I didn't know that the realization was coming, would slam me. I wasn't thinking about what would happen next.

I was just thinking that Cec wouldn't want anyone to see her like this. Her lips were dry and crusted, face tinged yellow. Her right eyelid hung open, as though she was trying to sneak a final peek. Her eyeballs had rolled heavenward as they had so often when she would disappear into one of her morphine-induced hallucinations. *My other world*, she called it.

I needed the others here with me. I needed them to help me believe this was really happening. I went to the door and opened it, to let Mom and Dad in. They looked at her and then at me, with a kind of shocked sadness.

One by one I called her family, and one by one they answered, none of them expecting this call tonight. She'd had a rough day, but she'd had rough days before. She'd been in extreme pain, but she'd been in pain before. I asked them to come, the ones who lived in the city, and they said they would. I called Lora first. "But I was just there," she said. Mom and Dad called Cor and Jer.

Please don't give me grief about this, Babe. Remember when Ellen died? Remember how you needed to see her?

Cec's room filled slowly. They entered quietly. Some with tears. I heard small gasps. They bent over her, touched cautiously, talked in whispers. They gave me hugs and asked how it had happened. I said I'd tell them later. The wastepaper basket filled with soggy tissues.

Lawrence brought plastic bags to put her belongings in.

Dad carried the bags out to the car.

One by one they said their final goodbyes then gathered in the hallway to wait for me, talking quietly.

She'll never be back, I thought to myself, trying to grasp what had just happened. So strange to see her lying flat on her back. This, to me, was the greatest indication that she was gone. She hadn't been able to lie flat for weeks.

I removed the chain with the cross from around her neck, and the rings from her fingers. Her skin was surprisingly cold to the touch. I lifted the sheet to look at her feet and legs, the bunion on her right foot and the big toe that curled sharply in, the swollen legs that I had shaved just the day before, and the swollen feet that I had massaged in the final hour.

I let the sheet fall. The backs of her ears were deepening purple, the blood gathering. All liquids had ceased coursing and were being pushed downward by gravity. I heard a faint gurgling sound from the back of her throat. The final sounds to escape her.

I had known, when her head fell forward. I'd watched her chest, waiting for a breath, a sigh, a flutter of eyelids.

Was her spirit still there then? Was she hovering? Did she hear me say, "I think she's gone"? Did she see me flee?

I was there until the end. I said I would be, and I was, with tremors of relief and panic.

Her hands now still, no longer able to wipe the tears from my face. I'd never again feel her fingers on the back of my neck.

I kissed her on the forehead, and again on the bruise under her eye. She didn't blink. She didn't move.

"Goodbye, Babe."

I pulled open the wide steel door. The conversations in the hallway stopped. All the faces turned to look at me. I kept my eyes on the floor as I pulled the door closed behind me. I heard the final click and thought to myself: *There. Now I never, ever have to do that again.*

No one would have blamed me if I'd said it out loud, not after the last two and half weeks and the horror of watching her suffer. They would have nodded. They would have thought they understood.

But what I really meant was the other agony—the solitary confinement of being alone with her, the unrelenting suffocation of her jealousy, her barbed disapprovals. Me trying to please and never succeeding. For eight and a half years. All of that finished.

I looked up. I nodded solemnly. Mom took my arm. We walked slowly down the hall. A procession.

Leo was at the nurse's station. I stopped to thank him.

It didn't feel right, walking out of the ward, leaving her behind. But the moment had come. I was free to leave. My face felt heavy. My steps were light.

Acknowledgements

Cease would never have come into being if Cecile Kaysoe hadn't walked into my life all those years ago. I am grateful to her for who she was, her unique way of looking at the world, her dry humor, even her sharp edges. She was right when she said that she would always be with me. She most certainly is.

There are many people who helped me with this book.

As *Cease* started to evolve from scattered bits of writing, I had the great fortune to receive input and guidance from Merilyn Simonds. She offered me a perceptive reading of multiple drafts and gave me much-needed perspective. Her insights, and the steadying hand of her guidance, were reliable and constant from the first draft right through to a fully realized manuscript. Thank you!

Aritha van Herk, sage counsel and friend, was my first writing instructor and gave me the writing "toolkit" that I still use today. Her mentorship has been invaluable, her badgering constructive, and her friendship a refuge. Contrary to what she claims, I do, in fact, listen to what she says and even follow her advice.

For her unwavering belief in me, a friendship that keeps on giving and for being consistently tuned in to my wavelength, a big thank you to Joanna Buhr.

Randal Macnair and Carolyn Nikodym of Oolichan

Books were both a true pleasure to work with. My appreciation goes to Randal for his thoughtful guidance and unflappable good humour. A special thank you to Carolyn for her long hours and unflagging patience, and also to Robyn Read for her judicious edit.

Thank you to Gail Corbett for being the kind of friend where long silences don't matter. To Penny Smallwood for listening and understanding. To Marilyn Elliott for being a kindred spirit and for writing her thoughts and responses as she was reading an early draft. To Rob McClement for coming back into my life. To the Tarpies for laughter, lamb chops and front row seats to Leonard. A special thank you to Carolynn Hoy for suggesting I contact Merilyn Simonds.

Thank you to Cec's family for your crazy sense of humour and unflagging support. To Shelly, Matt, Cail, Norma, Betty and David, thank you for staying in touch.

And most importantly, thank you to my family, and especially my mom and dad. I have lived my life with the rock solid certainty that if ever I needed anything and you could provide it, you would. Many times, you have. Thank you for being there, especially when the going got tough, and for always loving me.

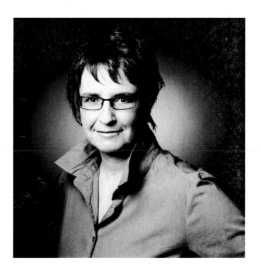

Lynette Loeppky was born and raised on the flat Manitoba prairie where the summer rain is always warm. After graduation from the University of Calgary with a BA she discovered an aptitude for sales and launched into a corporate sales career. Lynette has travelled extensively and lived for an extended time in Denmark, but counts amongst her greatest adventures the eight years that she and her partner Cecile tended an Old MacDonald-style hobby farm in southern Alberta. She now lives in Calgary with her dogs, Noddy and Charlie, who do an excellent job of getting her away from her computer and out into the elements on a daily basis. *Cease* is her first book.